Basic Principles of Ophthalmic Surgery

Anthony C. Arnold, MD, Executive Editor

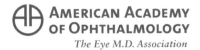

**AMERICAN ACADEMY
OF OPHTHALMOLOGY**
The Eye M.D. Association

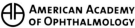
**AMERICAN ACADEMY
OF OPHTHALMOLOGY**
The Eye M.D. Association

P.O. Box 7424
San Francisco, CA 94120-7424

Clinical Education Secretaries
Thomas J. Liesegang, MD,
*Senior Secretary for
Clinical Education*

Gregory L. Skuta, MD,
*Secretary for Ophthalmic
Knowledge*

Academy Staff
Richard A. Zorab, *Vice President,
Ophthalmic Knowledge,
Clinical Education Division*
Hal Straus, *Director of Publications*
Kimberly Torgerson, *Publications
Manager*
Ruth Modric, *Production Manager*
Denise Evenson, *Design*
Nate Grant, *Executive Assistant*
Debra Marchi, *Administrative
Assistant*

The authors disclose the following financial relationships:

Anthony J. Aldave, MD: consultant fees, Allergan; grant support, National Eye Institute
Anthony C. Arnold, MD: consultant and lecture fees, Pfizer Ophthalmics
Steven J. Gedde, MD: lecture fees, Merck U.S. Human Health and Pfizer Ophthalmics
Jay M. Lustbader, MD: grant support, Alcon Laboratories, Inc; equity ownership/stock options, LCA Vision
Peter A. Quiros, MD: lecture fees, Allergan, Inc.
Nicholas J. Volpe, MD: consultant fees, Pfizer Ophthalmics
Norman Zabriskie, MD: lecture fees, Pfizer Ophthalmics

The other authors do not state significant financial interest or other relationship with the manufacturer of any commercial product discussed in the chapters that they contributed to this publication or with the manufacturer of any competing commercial product: Maria M. Aaron, MD; Keith D. Carter, MD; Madhuri Chilakapati, MD; Jack A. Cohen, MD, FACS; Oscar A. Cruz, MD; J. Paul Dunn, MD; Eric R. Holz, MD; Aaleya Koreishi, MD; Paul D. Langer, MD; Jennifer Lee, MD; Andrew G. Lee, MD; Yunhee Lee, MD, MPH; Casey Mickler, MS; Frank J. Moya, MD; Ensa K. Pillow, MD; Scott Sigler, MD; David K. Wallace, MD; Edward J. Wladis, MD.

Library of Congress Cataloging-in-Publication Data
Basic principles of ophthalmic surgery / Anthony C. Arnold, executive editor.
   p. ; cm.
   Includes bibliographical references and index.
   ISBN 1–56055–629–3 (soft cover)
   1. Eye—Surgery. I. Arnold, Anthony C.
   [DNLM: 1. Ophthalmologic Surgical Procedures. 2. Eye Diseases—surgery.
WW 168 B311 2006]
   RE80.B37 2006
   617.7'1—dc22   2006005983

Contributors

Maria M. Aaron, MD
Director of the Residency
    Program; Assistant
    Professor, Ophthalmology
Emory University
Atlanta, Georgia

Anthony J. Aldave, MD
Assistant Professor of
    Ophthalmology; Director,
    UCLA Eye and Tissue
    Bank
Jules Stein Eye Institute
Los Angeles, California

Keith D. Carter, MD
Medical Director,
    Ophthalmology Clinical
    Services; Director, Resident
    Education Program
University of Iowa Roy J.
    and Lucille A. Carver
    College of Medicine and
    UI Hospitals and Clinics
Iowa City, Iowa

Madhuri Chilakapati, MD
Fellow, Pediatric
    Ophthalmology and
    Strabismus
Cullen Eye Institute,
    Department of
    Ophthalmology, Baylor
    College of Medicine, and
    Texas Children's Hospital
Houston, Texas

Jack A. Cohen, MD, FACS
Associate Professor of
    Ophthalmology; Associate
    Chair for Education and
    Program Director
Rush University Medical
    Center
Chicago, Illinois

Oscar A. Cruz, MD
Professor and Chairman of
    Ophthalmology
St. Louis University School of
    Medicine
St. Louis, Missouri

J. Paul Dieckert, MD
Chief, Vitreoretinal Section;
    Professor, TAMUHSC;
    Chairman, Board of
    Directors; Chief of Staff,
    Scott and White Hospital
Temple, Texas

James P. Dunn, MD
Associate Professor of
    Ophthalmology; SOCA
    Clinical Director; Residency
    Education Director
The Wilmer Ophthalmological
    Institute
Baltimore, Maryland

Steven J. Gedde, MD
Associate Professor of
    Ophthalmology; Residency
    Program Director
Bascom Palmer Eye Institute
Miami, Florida

Eric R. Holz, MD
Associate Professor of
    Ophthalmology
Baylor College of Medicine
Houston, Texas

Aaleya Koreishi, MD
Baltimore, Maryland

Paul D. Langer, MD, FACS
Assistant Professor of
    Ophthalmology; Director,
    Division of Oculoplastics/
    Orbital Surgery; Director,
    Resident Training Program
New Jersey Medical School
Newark, New Jersey

Andrew G. Lee, MD
Professor of Ophthalmology,
    Neurology, and
    Neurosurgery
Department of
    Ophthalmology & Visual
    Sciences
University of Iowa Hospitals
    and Clinics
Iowa City, Iowa

Jennifer Lee, MD
Washington Pacific Eye
    Association
Kirkland, Washington

Yunhee Lee, MD, MPH
Assistant Professor of Clinical
    Ophthalmology; Medical
    Director; Division Chief
Bascom Palmer Eye Institute
    of the Palm Beaches
Miami, Florida

Jay M. Lustbader, MD
Professor and Chairman
Department of
    Ophthalmology
Georgetown University
    Hospital
Washington, DC

Casey Mickler, MS
St. Louis, Missouri

Frank J. Moya, MD
Assistant Consulting Professor
    of Ophthalmology,
    Glaucoma Service
Duke University Eye Center
Winston-Salem, North
    Carolina

Ensa K. Pillow, MD
Dean A. McGee Eye Institute
Oklahoma City, Oklahoma

Peter A. Quiros, MD
Assistant Professor
Department of
  Ophthalmology
University of Southern
  California
Doheny Eye Institute
Los Angeles, California

Scott C. Sigler, MD
Dean A. McGee Eye Institute
Oklahoma City, Oklahoma

Nicholas J. Volpe, MD
Director, Ophthalmology
  Residency Program; Vice
  Chairman Clinical Practice
Scheie Eye Institute
Philadelphia, Pennsylvania

David K. Wallace, MD
Associate Professor of
  Ophthalmology
Pediatric Ophthalmology &
  Strabismus
Duke University Eye Center
Durham, North Carolina

Edward J. Wladis, MD
Oculoplastics Fellow
Scheie Eye Institute
Philadelphia, Pennsylvania

Norman A. Zabriskie, MD
John Moran Eye Center
Salt Lake City, Utah

Contents

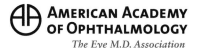
AMERICAN ACADEMY OF OPHTHALMOLOGY
The Eye M.D. Association

Dear Ophthalmology Resident and Program Director:

As part of the American Academy of Ophthalmology's ongoing commitment to resident education, we are underwriting the cost of *Basic Principles of Ophthalmic Surgery,* edited by Anthony C. Arnold, MD, so that it can be provided free of charge to first-year ophthalmology residents as part of the Basic Clinical and Science Course.

I hope that you will find the knowledge provided in these pages a useful adjunct to your education and that it will help you become a safe and proficient eye surgeon during your training over the next three years.

On behalf of the American Academy of Ophthalmology, I wish you success during your ophthalmology training and in your chosen career.

Sincerely,

H. Dunbar Hoskins, Jr., MD
Executive Vice-President
American Academy of Ophthalmology

Foreword

How do you teach surgery? How do you learn surgery? We surgeons have vivid memories of events in our surgical learning path—the first time we scrubbed in as medical students, the first time we sutured a laceration, or the first time we touched a beating heart—and many, many more.

As ophthalmologists, we remember the first successful cataract surgery and the patient's vision the next day—and we remember our first serious intraoperative complication and the steps we took to manage it. We likely shared a similar surgical learning process in residency training as we built on our general medical and surgical experience, sequentially adding knowledge, specific manual maneuvers, and procedural components through a combination of didactics, surgical "wet laboratories," observation, and supervised patient experience. Then, under supervision, we assembled it all as primary surgeon.

Is that the best way to learn surgery? Ultimately, no. Ultimately, skill acquisition will involve surgical simulator laboratories as well. They will permit the release of students to actual patient care only upon consistent technical competence and the deft management of common and uncommon but serious complications. The process will benefit surgeons in training and patients alike.

But surgery is much, much more than the technical performance of a set of skill components. A well-constructed set of surgical learning objectives must involve many subjects including the biomechanics of wound construction and healing, instrument design, surgical materials (such as sutures and irrigation fluids), and sterility and infection control. It should include patient selection, informed consent processes, medical ethics, postoperative management, and complication avoidance and management—among others.

For ophthalmology, surgery is a core and a complex competency, and education in this complex subject remains a process equally daunting for teacher and student alike. Anything that can facilitate the process benefits future patients.

In 2003 a group of those most responsible for the education of ophthalmology residents—the directors of ophthalmology residency training programs—determined that, although the ophthalmology literature is replete with surgical atlases, there was not an educational product aimed at the resident in training covering essential principles in ophthalmic surgery. For two years, a group of talented men and women under the leadership of Dr. Anthony C. Arnold have assembled the volume you have before you today.

Its objective is not to supplant the role of individual mentor-to-student surgical instruction, but to package many of the key elements of the surgical process and environment into an invaluable adjunct to the learning program. I believe they have succeeded, crafting a volume that should be on the desk of every resident.

As surgeons we have a profound obligation to our patients. They honor us by trusting to us their sight and sometimes their lives. This text acknowledges the scope and complexity of that obligation.

DAVID W. PARKE II, MD
President and Chief Executive Officer
Dean A. McGee Eye Institute
Oklahoma City, Oklahoma

Preface

The beginning ophthalmic surgeon faces the mastery of myriad new and complex skills, many of which have little carryover from prior medical education. The performance of surgery involves much more than the technical procedure itself. Skills needed encompass the full spectrum of surgical patient care, from patient selection to intraoperative techniques to postoperative management, and they are absolutely essential to the development of a competent surgeon.

There is very little available in the way of structured curricula to guide the ophthalmology resident in the acquisition of these skills. *Basic Principles of Ophthalmic Surgery* evolved in response to a request from the American Board of Ophthalmology to assist in improving training in ophthalmic surgical skills.

A core group of residency program directors directly involved in the education of residents collaborated to develop this book, ophthalmologists who rose to the challenge of creating a basic introduction to care of the ophthalmic surgical patient, while answering the simple everyday questions that the neophyte surgeon faces.

We hope that the book will prepare the resident to enter the realm of ophthalmic surgery with confidence. The book is composed of four parts:

- Part I covers evaluation and preparation, from patient selection to preparation of the patient and the surgeon.
- Part II introduces surgical instrumentation and materials, including surgical microscopes, surgical loupes, major categories of instruments and blades, and suture materials and needles.
- Part III presents an overview of seven specific aspects of surgery, from aseptic technique to an example of a specific surgical technique that the beginning surgeon may encounter—wound construction in cataract surgery.
- Part IV addresses postoperative considerations, including the healing process, dressings, and issues related to postoperative management.

Throughout, key points, self-assessment questions, photographs, and illustrations help reinforce learning.

Acknowledgments

This book has been reviewed and has been approved as a companion volume to the Academy's 13-volume *Basic and Clinical Science Course* (BCSC). The BCSC is the foundation course for residents and source of up-to-date clinical knowledge for practitioners. Thanks and appreciation go to the following BCSC Committee chairs for their helpful suggestions for this and future editions: Neil H. Atebara, MD; George A. Cioffi, MD; James C. Bobrow, MD; Louis B. Cantor, MD (Chair); K.V. Chalam, MD, PhD; John Bryan Holds, MD; Lanning B. Kline, MD; Ramana S. Moorthy, MD; Eric P. Purdy, MD; Edward L. Raab, MD; Carl Regillo, MD; James J. Reidy, MD, FACS; Debra J. Shetlar, MD; and Jayne S. Weiss, MD.

I am also grateful to Dr. David W. Parke II, MD, for his review of, and comments on, the initial drafts of the chapters and for agreeing to write the Foreword. The editorial and production expertise of Academy staff is deeply appreciated.

ANTHONY C. ARNOLD, MD
Professor and Chief, Division of Neuro-Ophthalmology
Director, UCLA Optic Neuropathy Center
Jules Stein Eye Institute
Department of Ophthalmology, University of California
Los Angeles, California

Part I

Evaluation and Preparation

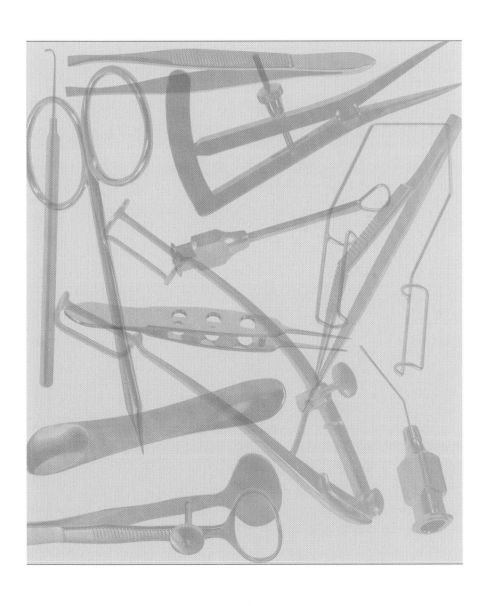

Chapter 1

Patient Selection

Maria M. Aaron, MD

The performance of surgery involves much more than the procedure itself. The beginning surgeon often focuses on the successful completion of the technical procedure—merely getting from point A to point B—without complications. Successful surgery, however, also requires careful patient selection, preoperative evaluation, and postoperative care. This chapter focuses on issues of patient selection, including criteria for surgical intervention, factors affecting surgical risk, ethical considerations including informed consent and advertising, and the implications of the surgeon's experience.

CRITERIA FOR SURGICAL INTERVENTION

The surgeon must carefully assess the patient's complaints and expectations for surgery. Upon reviewing the clinical pathology, he or she must determine if the surgical procedure will accomplish the desired outcome. For example, the patient with mild to moderate macular degeneration undergoing cataract extraction might be expecting a 20/20 result similar to that of others who have had the procedure; consequently, the surgeon must communicate a reasonable expectation of more limited visual acuity in this situation. Moreover, in a patient with severe macular degeneration, the surgical procedure might not be expected to benefit vision enough to justify cataract extraction at all.

In addition to understanding the patient's expectations, the surgeon must carefully review the clinical findings in order to accurately assess risk, evaluate whether surgery is justified, and communicate the risk-benefit ratio clearly

Table 1.1. Common Concerns to Consider Before Cataract Surgery

Condition	Risk
History:	
Previous trauma	Zonular weakness
General physical condition:	
Dementia	Altered response to anesthesia
	Movement during procedure
Severe spine/neck disease	Inability to lie supine
Congestive heart failure	Inability to lie supine
Anterior segment:	
Abnormally shallow anterior chamber	Reduction of working space
Abnormally deep anterior chamber	Difficulty with maneuvers
Exposure keratopathy	Corneal decompensation
Endothelial guttata	Corneal decompensation
History of iritis or inflammatory condition	Severe postoperative inflammation
Poor pupillary dilation	Challenging nuclear removal
	Iris Prolapse
Pseudoexfoliation	Poor dilation and zonular weakness
Advanced glaucoma	Spike in intraocular pressure
Prior trabeculectomy	Failure of shunt
Corneal scars	Poor visualization
Phacodonesis	Zonular weakness
Mature cataract or poor red reflex	Poor visualization of capsulorrhexis
Posterior segment:	
Previous pars plana vitrectomy	Loss of vitreous support
High myopia	Retinal detachment
Diabetic retinopathy	Progression of disease
Macular degeneration	Possible progression of disease
Other macular pathology	Limited visual outcome

to the patient. Careful clinical evaluation may reveal coexisting disease that might increase the potential risks of surgery. For example, a patient who has a moderate degree of corneal endothelial guttata who is undergoing phacoemulsification for a dense brunescent lens has the added risk of corneal decompensation. Table 1.1 lists common coexisting findings to consider when evaluating patients for cataract surgery, which is the type of surgery in which the beginning surgeon is most likely to be involved. While the implications of such abnormalities may vary depending upon the clinical situation and the experience of the surgeon, preoperative examination should include their consideration in every case.

FACTORS AFFECTING SURGICAL RISK

Ophthalmic surgical procedures are often performed on elderly patients who require careful medical evaluation to avoid surgical or systemic complications. While a patient's age does not necessarily correlate with his or her physical and mental status, older patients often have concomitant medical conditions requiring multiple medications. Proper preoperative medical assessment allows for selection of proper surgical candidates and helps ensure a smooth operative procedure and course in those who proceed to surgery.

Preoperative medical evaluation, either a brief survey by the surgeon, or a detailed assessment by a medical specialist, depending on the clinical situation, allows for selection of those patients who can safely undergo surgery and identification of those who either require medical care before surgery or who cannot safely proceed. The examiner should take a thorough history—including questions about medications, allergies, bleeding disorders and prior surgical procedures—during the preoperative assessment. He or she should also pay careful attention to a patient's use of aspirin-containing products and additional medications that may cause bleeding, including warfarin sodium (Coumadin), heparin, nonsteroidal anti-inflammatory drugs (NSAIDs), and herbal therapics such as Ginkgo biloba, garlic, and ginger. Many patients are unaware that aspirin and NSAIDs may cause bleeding and therefore do not report them unless specifically questioned. In patients requiring oral anticoagulants for prevention of stroke and transient ischemic attack, suspension of these agents carries risks, and alternative anesthesia or consultation with the patient's physician should be considered. Specific situations that may require special evaluation or therapy before surgery include cardiac disease, hypertension, pulmonary disease, and diabetes. Issues of anesthesia may be a concern with children and people with altered mental status.

Cardiac Disease

Patients with cardiac disease should be evaluated for any recent ischemic events, arrhythmias, or congestive heart failure (CHF). Patients with severe CHF may have difficulty lying supine for the duration of the procedure and may require intensive therapy to optimize cardiac status before surgery. (See

Chapter 2 for discussion of positioning the patient.) If the patient is unstable or if the surgeon has any degree of uncertainty about the cardiac stability, the cardiologist or primary care provider should clear the patient before the performance of the ophthalmic procedure.

Hypertension

Arterial blood pressure control is essential in patients undergoing ophthalmic surgery, as uncontrolled pressure increases risk of cardiovascular complications. Patients with a systolic blood pressure over 180 mmHg and diastolic over 100 mmHg should be evaluated and treated before the performance of an elective procedure.

Pulmonary Disease

The patient with severe chronic obstructive pulmonary disease or asthma will need clearance by his or her pulmonary or primary care physician before elective surgery. Optimization of pulmonary function reduces cardiopulmonary risks of anesthesia. Uncontrolled cough increases risk of complications in intraocular surgery, in both intraoperative and postoperative periods; patients with this condition require careful screening and management before consideration for surgery.

Diabetes

Optimal control of diabetes may reduce risks of general anesthesia and postoperative infection. Patients with uncontrolled diabetes should be evaluated and managed by a medical specialist before elective ophthalmic surgery.

Children

Children who have a family history of unexplained morbidity with anesthesia should be suspected of having a predisposition to malignant hyperthermia, a rare genetic disorder of skeletal muscle metabolism. Any such question should be addressed by the patient's medical and anesthesia team before surgery. Chapter 9 reviews symptoms of malignant hyperthermia; early recognition and action may be life-saving.

Altered Mental Status

Patients with altered mental function present specific problems in understanding the surgical procedure and postoperative conditions and may be unable to cooperate for surgery under local anesthesia. These patients require the participation of a family member in the preoperative, operative, and postoperative states. They also need additional consideration with regard to the choice of anesthesia (eg, general or local).

ETHICAL CONSIDERATIONS

Informed Consent

Chapter 2 reviews the details of the informed consent process. With regard to patient selection, however, three primary issues apply:

1. The surgeon has the responsibility to determine whether a patient is able to understand the nature of the procedure and potential risks, and then to make an autonomous decision whether to proceed. If the patient is unable to do so, or if uncertainty exists about his or her competence to make this decision, elective surgery should be deferred pending clarification of the issue (possibly with legal consultation). In some circumstances, a chosen surrogate may make the decision.
2. The patient has the right to make his or her own decisions regarding medical treatment, and he or she may contribute to the process of selection for surgery. For example, a moderate nuclear cataract in a patient with 20/50 vision may or may not require surgery. An airline pilot might desire that his or her cataract be removed, whereas an elderly person may feel comfortable continuing daily life with 20/50 vision.
3. The patient has the right to know that a resident in training will perform as the primary surgeon, with careful supervision by attending faculty. This must be explicitly explained during the consent process. Patient selection must take into account those who are uncomfortable with this situation, so that alternate planning for surgical care can be made.

Advertising

The fundamental principle in medical advertising is that communications to the public must be accurate. Before the 20th century, advertising for patient recruitment was prohibited because it was considered "derogatory to the dignity of the profession to resort to public advertisements." However, in 1977, it became unlawful for physicians to restrict advertising. With the recent explosion of refractive surgical procedures, the ethical concepts of advertising must be carefully considered. Care must be taken to portray all aspects of surgery accurately, without misleading the public, and to avoid claims of superiority or exclusivity that promote the physician's business rather than the patient's best interest. Similarly, one must avoid any patient education program or referral process that utilizes coercion to encourage surgery or limit patient options for surgical referral.

IMPLICATIONS OF THE SURGEON'S EXPERIENCE

The surgeon is responsible for assessing whether he or she has attained the level of experience required to perform specific surgical procedures. In residency training, the attending faculty generally sets guidelines and monitors them, with increasingly complex or difficult cases being assigned to more senior residents with greater surgical experience. Thus, the patient selection process includes assigning certain categories of surgical candidates to residents at the appropriate level of training. For example, in cataract surgery, cases that might be expected to present challenges at surgery (eg, patients who are monocular, have poor pupil dilation, poor visualization due to corneal disease, phacodonesis, or high myopia) are reserved for experienced surgeons. Similarly, patients who require surgery to be completed in the least amount of time (eg, those who have limited cooperation due to altered mental status or those with severe medical problems limiting tolerance for prolonged procedures) are assigned to the most experienced surgeons.

This principle also holds after the completion of residency training, as surgical technology advances and new techniques become available. Patients who are candidates for new techniques must be selected according to the expertise of the surgeon.

KEY POINTS

→ A thorough preoperative medical evaluation is essential in appropriate patient selection.

→ Patients with cardiac disease, hypertension, pulmonary disease, or diabetes may require special evaluation or therapy before surgery. Issues of anesthesia may be a concern with children and people with altered mental status.

→ Appropriate patient selection includes
  – Ensuring that indications for surgical intervention are appropriate and that the risk-benefit ratio is satisfactory
  – Carefully assessing medical risk factors and ensuring that the patient's general medical status is optimized prior to surgery
  – Ascertaining that the patient understands and agrees to the indications, risks, benefits, and alternatives for surgery
  – Avoidance of coercion in proceeding with surgery
  – Ensuring that the proposed surgical procedure is one for which the surgeon has adequate training and experience

SELF-ASSESSMENT TEST

1. Medications that may increase the risk of bleeding include
   a. Aspirin
   b. NSAIDs
   c. Coumadin
   d. All of the above
2. List at least three features that a preoperative medical evaluation should address.
3. The decision to recommend cataract surgery includes consideration of which of the following factors? (list all that apply)
   a. Coexistent macular disease
   b. Patient's visual requirements
   c. Coexistent corneal disease
   d. Family history of macular degeneration

For preferred responses to these questions, see pages 223–224.

SUGGESTED READING

American Academy of Ophthalmology. *Communications to the Public* [Advisory Opinion]. San Francisco: American Academy of Ophthalmology; 2003.

American Academy of Ophthalmology. *Ethical Ophthalmologist Series* [audio CDs]. San Francisco: American Academy of Ophthalmology.

American Academy of Ophthalmology. *Informed Consent* [Advisory Opinion]. San Francisco: American Academy of Ophthalmology; 2004.

Buratto L, Barboni P, Firrinicieli R. Developments in cataract surgery. In: Buratto L, Werner L, Zanini M, et al, eds. *Phacoemulsification. Principles and Techniques.* 2nd ed. Thorofare, NJ: Slack; 2003.

Feldman MA. The ophthalmic patient: medical assessment and management. In: Gottsch JD, Stark WJ, Goldberg MF, eds. *Rob & Smith's Operative Surgery: Ophthalmic Surgery.* 5th ed. New York, NY: Oxford University Press, Inc; 1999.

Parke DW, ed. Ethics and the American Academy of Ophthalmology. In: *The Profession of Ophthalmology: Practice Management, Ethics, and Advocacy.* San Francisco: American Academy of Ophthalmology; 2005:183–194.

Reiser SJ, Dyck AJ, Curran WJ, eds. *Ethics in Medicine: Historical Perspectives and Contemporary Concerns.* Cambridge: MIT Press; 1982.

Chapter 2

Preparation of the Patient

Madhuri Chilakapati, MD
Jack A. Cohen, MD, FACS

Appropriate preparation of a patient for surgery greatly impacts both the surgeon and the patient's entire surgical experience. Recognition of the importance of this process early in residency encourages the development of good habits seen in successful surgeons who maintain good rapport with their patients and effectively manage expectations. Patient preparation begins in the office and continues preoperatively in the operating room.

PREPARATIONS IN THE OFFICE

After the surgeon has assessed the patient and decided that surgery is a viable option, the next steps involve obtaining informed consent and scheduling the surgery. The essence of the informed decision-making process lies in effective physician–patient communication. The physician empowers the patient with the knowledge required to make an educated decision regarding medical care. At all times, the patient should feel in control of the decision-making process and able to decide what happens to his or her body.

Informed Consent

Chapter 1 introduced concepts of informed consent considered in selecting patients for surgery. Informed consent in preparing the patient for surgery develops from the patient's understanding of several elements.

These elements include the following:

→ The nature of the procedure
→ Reasonable alternatives to the proposed intervention
→ Explanation of the risks, benefits, and uncertainties related to each
  alternative
→ Assessment of the patient's understanding
→ Acceptance of the intervention by the patient

Procedure, Alternatives, and Risks

The depth of the discussion depends on the nature of the procedure and the number of risks, benefits, and alternatives. The American Academy of Oph-thalmology suggests that the content of this discussion should include what a "reasonable" patient would want to know. However, the difficulty in imple-menting a reasonable patient standard is also recognized because it involves determining what information is relevant for a particular patient. In most ophthalmic surgeries, the ultimate goals are to improve vision, preserve vision, or enhance appearance. The most common risks include infection, bleeding, loss of vision, scarring, and possible need for repeat surgery.

Discussion of alternatives should incorporate all options including medi-cal management and observation even if these choices are not ideal. Allow the patient to ask as many questions as necessary to facilitate comprehension of the intervention. This also enables the physician to assess the patient's under-standing of the procedure. Encourage patients to have family members present during the preoperative discussion so that they can provide support for the patient not only for the surgery itself, but during the decision-making process as well. Clearly outline any rehabilitation that will be needed after surgery and the average number of postoperative visits needed so the patient has an under-standing of the post operative course as well. Attention to these types of details helps ensure that adequate informed consent is obtained.

Discussion of the procedure should also include a description of anesthe-sia options. In ophthalmology, surgery may be performed with a variety of anesthetic techniques including topical, local, intravenous sedation, and general anesthesia (see Chapter 8). The physician should explain the preferred anes-thetic option for the procedure so that the patient knows what to expect and the physician can anticipate potential problems. A review of the medical his-tory and physical examination results will determine indications or contraindi-cations for specific anesthesia techniques. The anesthesia service determines the choice of anesthesia technique and informed consent process for anesthesia.

Assessment and Acceptance

Special situations to consider in the consent process include surgery for minors, incompetent individuals, and emergencies. With minors and incompetent individuals, the consent process occurs with the legal guardian. If there is no legal guardian, state laws provide guidance for the hierarchy of appropriate decision makers. If no surrogate decision maker exists or if the situation is emergent, the physician acts in the best interests of the patient until a surrogate is found. Legal standards in these situations may vary by state, and in any questionable case, counsel should be consulted before proceeding with surgery.

Medical Clearance

Medical clearance should be obtained from the patient's internist or family practitioner before surgery. Although routine preoperative laboratory testing has not been proven to increase the safety of cataract surgery, consideration may be given to such testing on the recommendation of the patient's physician or for specific requirements of the medical facility involved. Basic tests in this workup include a complete metabolic profile, a complete blood count, and an electrocardiogram. For patients undergoing general anesthesia, a chest x-ray is also recommended. The surgeon must ensure that all diagnostic test results are reviewed before surgery.

Additional common preoperative issues (eg, prophylaxis against endocarditis, managing anticoagulation, and medication interaction with herbal supplements) should be discussed and managed in conjunction with the patient's physician. The American Heart Association guidelines for prophylactic management of patients with cardiac valvular disease must be followed. Guidelines and quantification of risks for discontinuing anticoagulation have been published; typically anticoagulation is continued in patients at high risk for thromboembolism. Certain herbal supplements such as Ginkgo biloba and vitamin E increase the risk of bleeding in patients taking Coumadin and must be considered.

PROCESS IN THE OPERATING ROOM

Various chapters in this book discuss aspects of the surgical process. The following overview summarizes operative considerations with the focus on ensuring the patient's comfort (Chapter 7 reviews specific precautions that are necessary to ensure the safety of the patient during ophthalmic surgery).

Meeting the Patient

In the preoperative holding area, it is important that the patient see the surgeon. He or she may be the only familiar face among the many people that the patient will see during the surgical experience. This contact reassures the patient and provides an opportunity for any last-minute questions.

Marking the Incision Site

Many surgeons mark surgical incision sites in the holding area before any sedation is given. This confirms the surgical eye with the patient and avoids any confusion in the operating room. Surgery on the incorrect eye is the most feared but fortunately preventable medical error in the ophthalmic operating room (see Chapter 7).

Administering Medications

Review the history and physical report to ascertain any changes in the patient's health status. In cataract surgery and many retinal procedures, dilating drops will be administered in the preoperative holding area. Many surgeons also use preoperative topical antibiotic on the day of surgery or several days before surgery, although there is no consensus on which antibiotics to use and no studies show that this course prevents endophthalmitis. Some cataract surgeons apply topical anesthetic such as nonpreserved lidocaine jelly in the holding area with or without a device such as a Honan balloon to lower intraocular pressure.

Consider communicating any concerns or special requirements to the anesthesia service as soon as possible. For example, if the patient had problems with anesthesia during a prior surgical procedure, make sure the service is aware of this. If a local anesthetic block is needed, notify the anesthetist so the patient receives adequate sedation. Bear in mind that in many institutions, anesthesiology administers local anesthetic blocks so they need to be scheduled preoperatively.

Communicating With the Staff

Before the patient is brought back to the operating room, speak with the operating room staff to see whether they have any questions. If any special materials were ordered, verify that they are available. When doing cataract surgery, check that the correct intraocular lens has been set out for the procedure.

When the patient comes into the operating room, the circulating nurse verifies the patient's name, surgical procedure, surgical site, and medical allergies. Then, the bed is positioned in the most ideal location near the microscope to maximize viewing of the surgical eye (often the floor is marked to help guide the placement of the bed). If general anesthesia is required, positioning of the bed occurs after the patient is intubated. Positioning the patient's head on the bed and relative to the microscope is the foundation upon which the remainder of the surgery is built. When this is done incorrectly, every subsequent step of the procedure may become a challenge. When working under the microscope, the eye should be positioned so that it is parallel to the ground. The height of the bed should be adjusted to optimize surgeon comfort when looking under the microscope. When first learning to operate, check the positioning of the microscope by turning it on and looking through the oculars to assess whether the patient's placement is correct. This also serves to check if the microscope is functioning properly. (Chapter 4 discusses in detail the positioning of the microscope, patient, and surgeon.)

Ensuring the Patient's Comfort

Make sure the patient is comfortable. Operating rooms are often cold, and the patient may prefer an extra blanket. The nurse can provide support for the patient's back as needed by placing a blanket roll or foam log under the knees. Since many surgeries are done with topical anesthesia or intravenous sedation, wrist bracelets that attach to the bed rails are often employed to ensure that the patient does not attempt to touch her face. Taping the patient's head down is helpful in preventing head movement during surgery.

If a local anesthetic block is needed, it is best to do it after positioning the patient. After adequate intravenous sedation, the planned block can be administered. Typically, the nurse or the anesthetist holds the patient's head so it does not move during the block due to the noxious stimulus. Taping of the head should occur after the block so the head can be placed in the most comfortable position for the block. The surgical prep and draping follow final positioning of the patient (see Chapter 8 for information about surgical prep and draping).

KEY POINTS

→ In providing informed consent to the patient, the surgeon must explain the nature of the procedure, reasonable alternatives to the proposed intervention, and the risks, benefits, and uncertainties related to each alternative.

→ Medical clearance for surgery includes assessment of cardiopulmonary status, anticoagulants, and antiplatelet agents. Clearance should be coordinated with the patient's primary care physician.

→ In the operating room, the surgeon is responsible for meeting and reassuring the patient, supervising preoperative ophthalmic medications, coordinating with anesthesia and nursing staff, and ensuring proper positioning and comfort of the patient.

SELF-ASSESSMENT TEST

1. The informed consent process (list all that apply)
   a. Consists of the preoperative counseling session alone
   b. Involves discussion of risk, benefit, and alternatives of surgery
   c. May be delegated to be performed by the surgical nurse
   d. Discourages consideration of alternatives to surgery that the surgeon feels are less appropriate

2. Preoperative medical preparation of the patient (list all that apply)
   a. Is not the surgeon's responsibility
   b. Requires chest x-ray, EKG, urinalysis, and CBC
   c. Requires discontinuing anticoagulants
   d. Is best performed in conjunction with the patient's primary physician if medical conditions coexist

3. Preparing the patient in the operating room includes attention to (list all that apply)
   a. Communication with the patient
   b. Head position
   c. Back and knee support
   d. Stability (control of hands and head)
   e. Comfortable temperature
   f. All of the above

For preferred responses to these questions, see pages 223–224.

SUGGESTED READING

American Academy of Ophthalmology. *Informed Consent* [Advisory Opinion]. San Francisco: American Academy of Ophthalmology; 2004.

Dajani AS, Taubert KA, Wilson W, et al. Prevention of bacterial endocarditis: recommendations by the American Heart Association. *JAMA*. 1997;277:1794–1801.

Kearon C, Hirsh J. Management of anticoagulation before and after elective surgery. *N Engl J Med*. 1997;336:1506–1511.

Liesegang TJ. Perioperative antibiotic prophylaxis in cataract surgery. *Cornea*. 1999;18:383–402.

Parke DW, ed. Ethics in ophthalmology. In: *The Profession of Ophthalmology*. San Francisco: American Academy of Ophthalmology; 2005:183–247.

Chapter 3

Preparation of the Surgeon

Eric R. Holz, MD

A great body of literature addresses ophthalmic surgical management, including details of surgical techniques, preparation of the patient, management of the operating theater, and postoperative care (aspects of these topics are discussed elsewhere in this book). Very little, however, has been written about preparation of the surgeon. The surgeon's ability to attain peak performance is clearly a key element in obtaining optimal surgical outcomes. Thorough familiarity with the patient, procedure, and operating room environment are the foundation of preparation. Other considerations include physical factors affecting the surgeon, handwashing, and control of the operating room environment. This chapter serves as a guide to creating a personalized routine for your own preparation as a surgeon. The development of good habits through repetition limits stress and anxiety and prepares the physician to perform to optimum potential.

FAMILIARIZATION

Chapters 1 and 2 discussed aspects of becoming familiar with the patient, deciding that surgery is the best option, and preparing the patient for surgery. In summary, several elements are important in the physician's interaction with his or her patient:

1. The surgeon should fully examine the patient preoperatively. This evaluation consists of a complete examination, including best-corrected

visual acuity measurement, a review of pertinent ancillary testing, and directed systemic evaluation. Review of ancillary testing may include IOL calculation data, fluorescein angiography, or neuroimaging such as MRI films.

2. A discussion ensues in order to understand the patient (especially reactions and concerns), educate the patient, answer questions, and obtain informed consent.

3. A surgical plan evolves during the preoperative examination. Clearly, first meeting a patient on a gurney in the operating room is ill advised. Delegating preoperative evaluation and management to technicians, optometrists, and colleagues is another practice to avoid if you are to be optimally prepared.

Understanding the Planned Procedure

Knowledge of the anticipated surgical procedure is an essential part of the familiarization process. As noted in Chapter 1, the surgeon is responsible for assessing whether he or she has attained the level of experience required to perform specific surgical procedures. Ideally, the beginning surgeon is prepared through the mentored experiences provided during ophthalmology residency training. Established techniques continue to evolve and new techniques are employed, and these developments require the surgeon's continuing education. On an ongoing basis, long after the completion of residency training, the surgeon must ensure that he or she is facile in all aspects of a proposed procedure; if knowledge gaps or uncertainties exist, the surgeon has the responsibility to arrange for consultation with and possible intraoperative assistance from an expert in the field.

Knowing Your Tools

Familiarity with the overall operating room environment is also crucial to preparation of the surgeon. Ophthalmic surgical instrumentation and machinery, including the phacoemulsification and vitrectomy units, are increasingly complex, and the surgeon needs to understand their inner workings in detail. Detailed discussion of surgical instrumentation and machinery is beyond the scope of this book. Equipment company representatives and other experienced surgeons are valuable sources of information in this area. (See Chapter 5 for an introduction to surgical instruments and blades.)

Consider performing a "dry run," including opening up surgical packs, setting up the machine, running through machine settings, and familiarizing yourself with the foot pedals and handpieces. The properly prepared surgeon knows the equipment better than the nursing staff! In cases of equipment malfunction or requirement for special measures, the surgeon's ultimate responsibility is to manage the situation correctly. In addition, an important, but frequently overlooked, area involves the location of items in the room. The physician is advised to go to the operating room during down time and go through each drawer and cabinet with the nursing staff. The location of suture material, intraocular lenses, non-set surgical instruments, and so on should be identified so that the surgeon is prepared to give instructions when the primary nurse is unavailable, particularly during after-hours cases.

PHYSICAL FACTORS AFFECTING THE SURGEON

A multitude of factors affect a physician's preparedness to perform surgery. Two of the commonly discussed physical factors are exercise and sleep deprivation. Physical exertion before surgery, involving as few as 20 knee bends, has been shown to significantly increase hand tremor when performing microsurgical tasks. This supports widely held beliefs that strenuous exercise, particularly upper-body weight lifting, should be avoided the day before and the day of surgery.

The relationship between sleep deprivation and physician performance has been studied superficially. Conclusions have been reached that "patient care may be compromised if a fatigued, sleep-deprived clinician is allowed to operate, administer an anesthetic, manage a medical crisis, or deal with an unusual or cognitively demanding clinical presentation." There is controversy regarding performance of particular activities but in general there is more degradation on tasks of longer duration requiring vigilance. Performance of longer, repetitive surgery may be more severely affected by sleep deprivation. Avoidance of physical exertion and a good night's sleep are important components in the preparation of the surgeon.

Substance Use or Abuse

Both legal and illicit drug use can affect surgical performance and the prepared surgeon understands their impact. It is obvious that physicians impaired by alcohol or illicit drugs should never operate; however, the use of caffeine and beta blockers has been an area of controversy.

Many doctors routinely drink coffee or tea before performing surgery, yet studies involving hand steadiness support the assertion that caffeine increases hand tremor. One study noted that after ingestion of 200 mg of caffeine, tremor was significantly increased when measured with a handheld laser pointer model. Another study, employing a high-resolution, noncontact position tracking system, found that ingestion of 200 mg of caffeine caused a 31% increase in tremor from baseline. Based on these data, caffeine should be avoided to minimize tremor during ocular surgery.

Performance artists and surgeons have employed β-adrenergic blocking drugs to improve their performance. Several studies assess the effect of β-blockers on ocular surgery, or hand tremor. Using the same high-resolution, noncontact position tracking system as employed for the caffeine study, subjects who ingested 10 mg of propranolol (a nonselective β-blocking agent) were found to have 22% less tremor than at baseline. No adverse effects or side effects were reported. Ophthalmology residents given 40 mg of propranolol 1 hour before performing ophthalmic microsurgery experienced a significant reduction in tremor and perceived anxiety. However, there was no difference in complication rates or difficulties during surgery. Similarly no negative effects or side effects were encountered in study participants. A study involving ingestion of timolol 12.5 mg as well as a postural orthotic concluded that neither "accorded a significant benefit in allaying hand tremor." In summary, β-blocker use, particularly oral propranolol, may diminish hand tremor, but this difference has not been proven to affect surgical outcomes.

HAND PREPARATION

Handwashing or scrubbing is a time-honored routine in surgery. Without question, handwashing decreases the surgeon's skin flora counts, which may in turn lower postoperative infection rates, especially in the event of glove failure. Several areas of controversy surround the surgical scrub, however. The duration of handwashing has been studied, with results indicating that a 2-minute period of chlorhexidine use is equivalent to 4- and 6-minute time periods. Improved alcohol solutions for handrubbing have become popular and are present in most institutions. A study reported that the use of a 75% aqueous alcoholic solution containing propanol-1, propanol-2, and mecetronium etilsulfate causes no difference in postoperative infection rates compared with use of 4% povidone iodine or 4% chlorhexidine gluconate. Additionally, handrubbing with an alcohol-based solution has been shown to result in a significantly lower skin flora count than handwashing with antiseptic soap during routine patient care.

In light of these findings, preparation of the hands for surgery should consist of a 2-minute scrubbing with chlorhexidine or povidone iodine or simple handwashing with soap followed by handrubbing with an appropriate alcohol-based solution. Generally accepted practice for the first scrub of the day includes a total duration of 5 minutes. Chapter 8 reviews the steps in the surgical hand scrub as well as the steps for gowning and gloving after the wash is complete.

OPERATING ROOM ENVIRONMENT

The surgeon must be able to give his or her full attention and concentration to the patient and the procedure. Preparation of the environment before surgery is an important step in minimizing distractions. Ideally the physician should clear his or her schedule a bit before and after surgery to avoid potential conflicts. Having to run to clinic or to another hospital creates significant stress and is suboptimal. Likewise, during surgery, minimize interruptions by telephone calls and pages or avoid them altogether.

Giving forethought to ergonomic issues is a simple, but often overlooked, element. A few minutes spent before the procedure to adjust the bed height, microscope (eyepiece pupillary distance, power, and centration), and wrist rest result in greater comfort and less stress for the surgeon. (Chapter 4 reviews these adjustments in detail.) Additionally, speaking with the scrub nurse and circulating nurse before the case allows them to anticipate your needs and to have readily available the necessary equipment and instruments. Simple communication before the surgery makes the team in the room more involved, understanding, and efficient; and as a result, the case runs more smoothly.

What About Music?

A frequent component of the operating room environment is music. Although music may relax the surgeon, staff, and patient, it should not be allowed to become a distraction. The musical selection, choice of compact disc, or radio station should be prepared before the surgical scrub. Volume and static should be checked and refined before surgery in order to avoid distractions while changing volume, stations, or discs.

KEY POINTS

→ Preparation of the surgeon includes detailed review of the patient's ophthalmologic and general medical status along with the planned surgical procedure.

→ The operating surgeon should become familiar with the complex equipment to be used in the procedure, including setup, positioning, and common malfunction remedies.

→ Sleep deprivation, physical exertion, and caffeine ingestion may all have a detrimental effect on a surgeon's performance.

SELF-ASSESSMENT TEST

1. In preparation for surgery, the surgeon (list all that apply)
   a. Need not necessarily examine the patient personally
   b. Must be facile with all steps of the planned procedure
   c. Should be familiar with all major equipment involved, including common causes of malfunction and their correction
   d. Should review all pertinent ancillary tests personally
2. List two physical factors that may negatively affect surgical performance.
3. The caffeine contained in one cup of coffee may induce detrimental hand tremor. (true or false)
4. The controversy in surgical hand preparation includes (list all that apply)
   a. Duration of scrub
   b. Composition of the antibacterial agent
   c. Necessity to scrub
   d. Requirement for gloves

For preferred responses to these questions, see pages 223–224.

SUGGESTED READING

Arnold RW, Springer DT, Engel WK, et al. The effect of wrist rest, caffeine, and oral timolol on the hand steadiness of ophthalmologists. *Ann Ophthalmol.* 1993;25:250–253.

Elman MJ, Sugar J, Fiscella R, et al. The effect of propranolol versus placebo on resident surgical performance. *Trans Am Ophthalmol Soc.* 1998;96:283–294.

Girou E, Loyeau S, Legrand P, et al. Efficacy of handrubbing with alcohol based solution versus standard handwashing with antiseptic soap: randomized clinical trial. *BMJ.* 2002;325:362–367.

Holmes JM, Toleikis SC, Jay WM. The effect of arm exercise and ocular massage on postural hand tremor. *Ann Ophthalmol.* 1992;24:156–158.

Humayun MU, Rader RS, Pieramici DJ, et al. Quantitative measurement of the effects of caffeine and propranolol on surgeon hand tremor. *Arch Ophthalmol.* 1997;115:371–374.

Lubahn JD, Dickson BG, Cooney TE. Effect of timolol versus a postural orthotic on hand tremor during microsurgery. *Microsurgery.* 2002;22:273–276.

Mürbe D, Hüttenbrink KB, Zahnert T, et al. Tremor in otosurgery: influence of physical strain on hand steadiness. *Otol Neurotol.* 2001;22:672–677.

O'Shaughnessy M, O'Malley VP, Corbett G, et al. Optimum duration of surgical scrub-time. *Br J Surg.* 1991;78:685–686.

Parienti JJ, Thibon P, Heller R, et al. Handrubbing with an aqueous alcoholic solution versus traditional surgical hand-scrubbing and 30-day surgical site infection rates: a randomized equivalence study. *JAMA.* 2002;288:722–727.

Parke DW, ed. Ethics in ophthalmology. In: *The Profession of Ophthalmology.* San Francisco: American Academy of Ophthalmology; 2005.

Samkoff JS, Jacques CH. A review of studies concerning effects of sleep deprivation and fatigue on residents' performance. *Acad Med.* 1991;66:687–693.

Weinger MB, Ancoli-Israel S. Sleep deprivation and clinical performance. *JAMA.* 2002;287:955–957.

Part II

Surgical Instrumentation and Materials

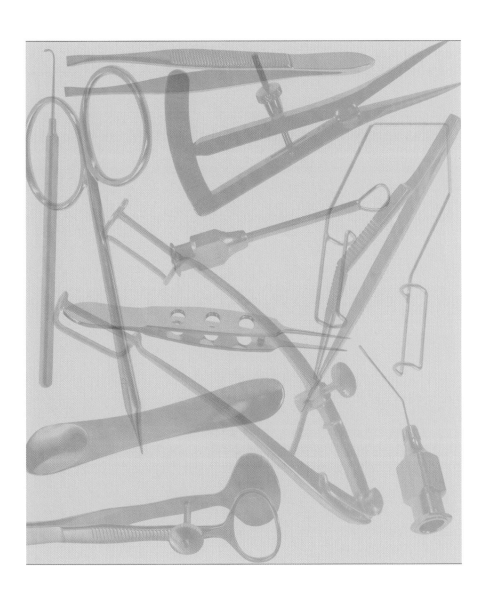

Chapter 4

The Operating Microscope and Surgical Loupes

Norman A. Zabriskie, MD

The development of the surgical microscope has revolutionized ophthalmic surgery. Historically, cataract surgery was performed without magnification. The modern surgical microscope makes possible the current standard of small-incision phacoemulsification with capsulorrhexis, complete nuclear and cortical removal, preservation of the posterior capsule, and in-the-bag placement of a foldable intraocular lens. Most retinovitreous surgical procedures are wholly dependent on the high magnification, lighting, and depth perception that the microscope affords. Surgical loupes provide magnification as well, with advantages and disadvantages when compared with the microscope. This chapter describes the practical use of both instruments in the operating room.

Just as a smooth cataract operation depends on the successful completion of a series of maneuvers in their proper order, maximal benefit from the operating microscope is obtained by repeating certain steps carefully and effectively each and every time. These include proper positioning of the patient and surgeon, hand positioning that reduces tremor, and efficient operation of the microscope.

ADVANTAGES AND DISADVANTAGES OF MAGNIFICATION

The many advantages of the modern-day surgical microscope may seem intuitive. Its lighting is excellent and uniform throughout the field and a good red reflex is usually readily obtained. Newer illumination systems can even enhance the red reflex in difficult cases such as those with small pupils. The light intensity is adjustable and filters protect the patient and surgeon from phototoxic effects. The optical system provides the surgeon with an excellent binocular wide-field stereoscopic view. Most microscopes can provide a stereoscopic view through an assistant arm as well, usually by way of a beam-splitter that splits the light between the surgeon and the assistant, usually in a 70/30 ratio. However, the newest microscopes can provide 100% stereo and 100% illumination to both the surgeon and the assistant via independent light sources. Such an advancement is particularly useful for teaching institutions where residents perform surgery while staff supervisors observe through the assistant arm of the microscope.

Magnification itself is obviously a significant advantage in ophthalmic surgery, but the control and variability of this magnification are the key benefits. Most microscopes offer a range of magnification from approximately 10 × to 30 × and foot pedal controls. Thus, the surgeon can focus on the posterior capsule and then into the anterior chamber, or from the mid-vitreous to the retinal surface, with a simple touch of the foot pedal. Motors on the microscope also provide motion control of the optical system in the x-y axis. This allows adjustment of the microscope to compensate for minor patient movements that change the operating axis.

The benefits of the microscope far outweigh the disadvantages, but several disadvantages are worth mentioning. Because of the high magnification, even the slightest vibration can disturb the view through the microscope. Operating rooms that house surgical microscopes must be constructed to very high vibration-dampening standards. Even maintenance or construction in adjacent rooms or floors can cause excessive vibration. In such cases it is not uncommon to have to search out the source of the vibration, usually a construction or maintenance worker, and have them stop their work until completion of a surgical case. High magnification also places greater demands on the surgeon. Any hand tremor or surgical misstep is magnified along with the ocular tissues. Controlling tremor and nerves can be more difficult in such a setting. This is particularly true for the beginning surgeon.

Another disadvantage of the operating microscope is that procedures requiring the surgeon to view the surgical field from multiple angles are not easily performed. Fortunately, surgical loupes provide a good alternative because of the flexibility of their viewing angle. In addition, loupes provide magnification that is well suited to many oculoplastic and strabismus surgeries, as well as scleral buckle surgery. The main disadvantage of loupes is their fixed focal length, which results in a fixed working distance for the surgeon.

PATIENT POSITIONING

Good patient positioning is essential for proper use of the surgical microscope. The goals of patient positioning, as related to the microscope, are to (1) maximize the view of the surgical field, especially the red reflex, (2) minimize the need for microscope adjustment during surgery, (3) allow good patient fixation on the microscope light for procedures under topical anesthesia, and (4) avoid excess light exposure to the patient.

Careful positioning of the surgical eye relative to the microscope is the first step in a successful surgery. Position the patient so that the corneal surface of the operative eye is parallel to the floor (Figure 4.1). This recommendation holds whether the surgical approach is temporal or at the 12:00 position, and whether using retrobulbar or topical anesthesia. Positioning the eye surface parallel to the floor is most easily accomplished if the surgical bed has a separate head rest with its own adjustment system (Figure 4.2). Usually one can

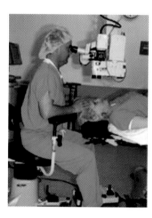

Figure 4.1. Good patient positioning with the "eye parallel to the floor." This maximizes the view for the surgeon and allows the patient to better fixate on the microscope light.

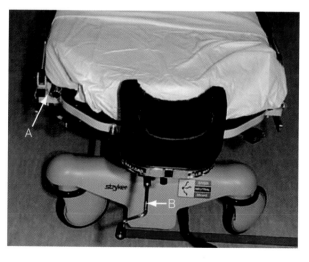

Figure 4.2. Outpatient surgical bed. Bed with separate head rest and independent head rest controls. Lever A controls the vertical position of the head rest and lever B changes the tilt of the head rest.

adjust both the tilt and the vertical position of the head rest without affecting the patient's overall position. With this flexibility, the surgeon can be very precise in adjusting the head of the patient even when anatomic challenges, such as kyphosis, might make proper positioning very difficult on a traditional operating room bed.

Having the surgical eye parallel to the floor is very important for proper use of the microscope, especially for topical anesthetic procedures. Such positioning allows the eye to be centered between the upper and lower eyelids when the patient fixates on the microscope light. This maximizes the quality of the surgical view as well as the red reflex, and it helps the patient to maintain proper fixation on the microscope light. If the patient is positioned so that her chin is up (Figure 4.3) and the superior limbus of the eye tilts toward the floor, fixation on the microscope light by the patient drives the eye toward the lower lid which can hinder the surgical view and the red reflex. Conversely, if the patient is in the chin-down position, with the inferior limbus tilting toward the floor, fixation on the microscope light drives the eye toward the upper lid, causing similar problems (Figure 4.4). This latter problem is particularly true

Figure 4.3. The chin-up patient position. This posture drives the eye to the lower lid when the patient fixates the microscope light.

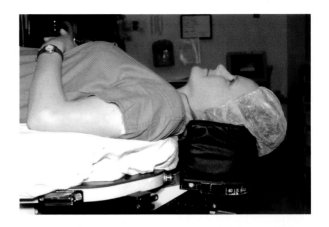

Figure 4.4. The chin-down patient position. This position drives the eye to the upper eyelid. This is a particularly troublesome position for a right-handed surgeon operating on a left eye from the temporal approach.

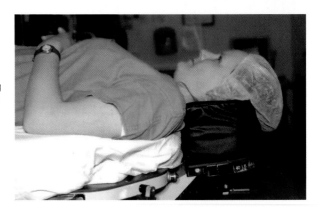

for a right-handed surgeon performing cataract surgery on a left eye from a temporal approach; the chin-down patient position must be avoided in this case. Failure to position the patient far enough onto the head rest is a common cause of the chin-down position. Before starting, make sure that the patient is fully onto the head rest. This will not only result in better patient positioning for surgery, but also greater comfort for the patient since the head and neck are much better supported.

Pearls and Pitfalls of Patient Positioning

If the patient is positioned properly at the start of the case, then any subsequent movement of the eye out of the surgical field is unwanted and the cause should be ascertained and corrected. In most cases, excessive movement of the operated eye is due to improper hand position by the surgeon, a point to be discussed later; however, sometimes the patient simply moves. If the case is being performed under topical anesthesia, the patient may have just lost fixation of the microscope light. A gentle reminder from the surgeon to "look at the light" or "find the light" will correct this problem. However, if after refixation on the microscope light, the upper lid still partly obscures the surgical eye, the patient has probably dropped her chin, and if covered by the lower lid, the patient has lifted her chin. The surgeon need simply ask the patient to "lift your chin" or "drop your chin," and the problem is corrected.

The surgical eye moving away from the surgeon characterizes another very common positioning problem during surgery from the temporal approach. For example, if the surgeon operates on a left eye temporally from the 3:00 position, the eye may move to the 9:00 position, and the surgeon repeatedly uses the x-y control on the foot pedal to move the microscope in that direction and center the image. Although this is usually due to the surgeon displacing the eye nasally with improper hand position, there is also a common tendency for the patient to rotate his head away from the temporal incision site. To correct this head rotation, either ask the patient to rotate his head back toward the surgeon, or you can take your nondominant hand and gently rotate the head back toward you in a very slow and controlled fashion. The latter approach is safer and more effective. Some patients have such a strong tendency to roll away from the incision site that the surgical assistant or scrub nurse must hold the patient's head in place.

Some patients are not able to lie flat. This may be due to difficulty breathing in the supine position, dizziness, or the patient's body habitus, including obesity and spinal kyphosis. One strategy for such patients is to elevate the head of the bead to about 30°. Raise the entire bed, and then use the reverse

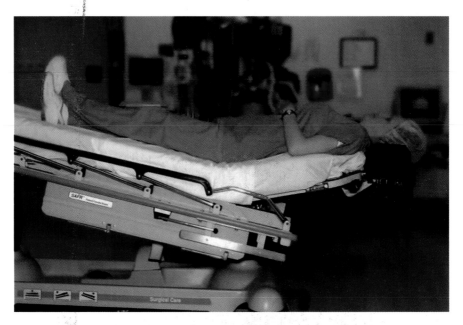

Figure 4.5. The patient unable to lie flat can be successfully positioned using this strategy. The head of the bed is elevated, the bed is raised, and then a reverse Trendelenburg position places the eye properly for the microscope.

Trendelenburg pedal to lower the head into position (Figure 4.5). This method maintains the 30° angle of the patient, while putting the head flat and into position for the microscope. This V-position reduces the patient's sensation of being in a completely flat position and therefore results in better tolerance and cooperation with the surgery. This method also works well for patients who are significantly kyphotic, in whom the head seems to dangle in midair above the head rest when the patient is placed in the supine position. This maneuver brings the head into contact with the head rest and allows good "eye parallel to the floor" positioning.

Infants and small children can pose unique positioning problems. Due to anesthesia requirements, these cases are often performed in main hospital operating rooms, on traditional surgical beds without separate head rests and independent controls. The main problem stems from the fact the infant head is bigger in proportion to the body than in adults, resulting in an exaggerated chin-down position. A shoulder roll, usually a rolled towel of appropriate size, placed under the child's shoulders extends the neck and places the head in the "eye parallel to the floor" position. The microscope can then be positioned as usual. This method can also be used in adults when a surgical bed with independent head rest controls is not available.

SURGEON POSITIONING

Proper positioning of the surgeon in relationship to the microscope allows easy control of the microscope foot pedal without disturbing the surgical field and maintains the surgeon's comfort throughout the case. Most forms of intra-ocular surgery that use an operating microscope are performed with the surgeon sitting at the head of the patient. The patient's bed must be raised enough to let the surgeon's legs slide under the patient's head. This can be thought of as placing the head of the patient in the lap of the surgeon. This assures that when the microscope is brought into position directly over the patient, the surgeon neither has to lean too far forward or back to view through the microscope oculars. This positioning promotes surgeon comfort during the case and places the surgeon's hands in the most ergonomically favorable position.

The microscope pedal is positioned to allow manipulation by the foot without altering the position of the surgical field. With the surgeon at the 12:00 position, the microscope pedal can be placed slightly to the side of the patient and the table. A second control pedal, for example one controlling a vitrectomy unit, can be placed at the other side. The surgeon's legs are then not directly under the bed itself and therefore it is easy to use the pedals without inadvertently bumping the surgical table and changing the position of the surgical field (Figure 4.6).

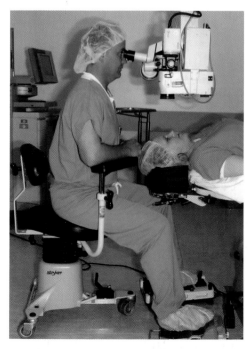

Figure 4.6. Surgeon positioning at the 12:00 position. The pedals are positioned just to the side of the patient and table. At the 12:00 position, it is relatively easy for the surgeon to avoid inadvertent contact with the overlying table.

The Temporal Approach

Proper surgeon positioning for the temporal approach is more difficult. As with other approaches, the surgeon's legs need to be far enough under the head of the patient. This again ensures that the surgeon has good ergonomic posture, without leaning too far forward or back. The challenge comes in placing the control pedals for the microscope and phacoemulsification unit. At the temporal position, one leg of the surgeon will be directly under the surgical bed. For example, when operating on the right eye of a patient from the temporal approach, the right leg of the surgeon is completely under the bed (Figure 4.7); temporal surgery on a left eye places the left leg in a similar position, with difficulty keeping the leg clear of the table (Figure 4.8). This is especially difficult for the taller surgeon. In the temporal approach, as compared with the 12:00 position, the bed must be raised to accommodate the surgeon's legs.

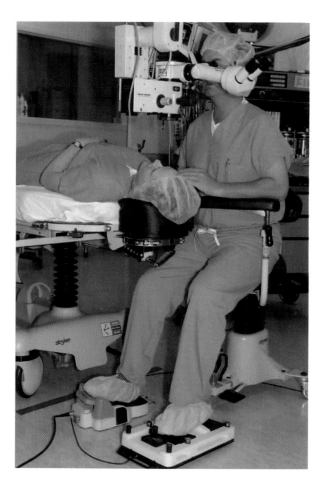

Figure 4.7. Surgeon positioning while operating on a right eye at the temporal position. Note that the right leg is completely under the surgical bed.

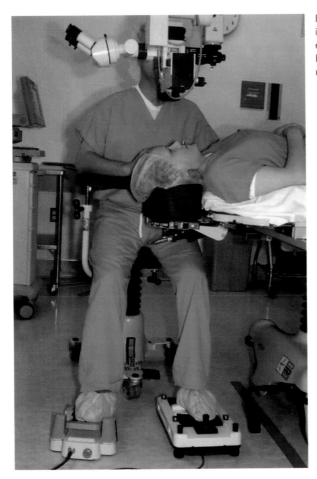

Figure 4.8. Surgeon positioning while operating on a left eye at the temporal position. Here, the left leg is completely under the surgical bed.

Because the bed must be higher, the microscope must be raised to allow proper focus; however, the surgeon's chair cannot be raised the same amount or again the surgeon will bump the bottom of the table. Thus, the surgeon must assume a quite erect torso posture to reach the oculars of the microscope. This can be particularly true for a surgeon with a short torso relative to leg length. However, as discussed later in this chapter, this erect torso posture is an important step in stabilizing the hands.

Pearls and Pitfalls of Surgeon Positioning

In summary, good positioning starts by making sure that the surgeon's body is sufficiently under the head of the patient. This is true at either the 12:00 or temporal position. If the surgeon does not get close enough to the patient, and the head of the patient does not overlie at least the knees and perhaps the thighs of the surgeon, the surgeon must lean too far forward to reach the microscope oculars. This is uncomfortable for the surgeon and extends the arms away from the body, which makes it more difficult to stabilize the hands. In the proper surgeon position relative to the patient, the surgeon will have an erect torso posture with a slight forward lean at the waist to reach the microscope oculars.

POSITIONING THE BED

The most common positioning error the beginning surgeon makes, when operating from the temporal position, is failing to raise the bed high enough. This is not a problem at the head of the patient, since at the 12:00 position the surgeon's legs are not under the surgical bed when controlling the foot pedals. However, as mentioned before, in the temporal position one leg has to be under the table. This creates a problem when the bed is not high enough and during pedal maneuvers, the surgeon bumps the underside of the table with his or her leg. This action elevates the bed slightly (Figure 4.9) and, under high microscopic magnification, causes the surgical field to go in and out of focus.

The bumping action can be a major problem for the beginning surgeon. It is far more common while controlling the microscope pedal than the phacoemulsification unit pedal, as the latter requires a downward motion on the foot pedal, lowering the knee and avoiding contact with the surgical bed. The microscope pedal, on the other hand, requires a rocking motion with the foot as the focus tab is controlled with the toe and the zoom tab is controlled with the heel. When the foot is flat on the pedal, both the toe down position controlling the focus tab and the heel down position required for the zoom tab elevate the knee, and it is during these maneuvers that the bed is most likely to be bumped.

Three steps help you avoid this problem:

1. Initially determine the proper bed height so that your legs may slide comfortably under the patient's head.
2. Make sure that the clearance is still adequate when your feet are on the pedals. Commonly, beginning surgeons set the bed height with their feet flat on the floor. Then when the feet are placed on the pedals, the bed is obviously too low.
3. If the microscope pedal is the one directly under the patient, rock your foot back and forth, controlling the focus and the zoom respectively,

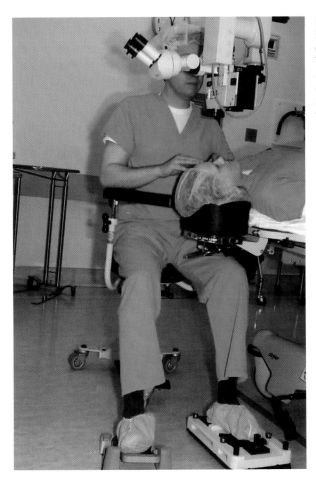

Figure 4.9. In this case, the left leg of the surgeon is in contact with the overlying bed. This creates a problem as the surgeon's leg elevates the bed during foot pedal maneuvers and defocuses the surgical field.

and assure proper clearance. It is also common for the beginning surgeon to have the leg extended all the way to the joystick of the pedal when setting the bed height. Once the case starts, and the surgeon has to bring the foot back to use either the focus or zoom tabs, the knee elevates dramatically and the bed is disturbed.

For surgeons with a relatively short torso, or long legs, it can sometimes be a challenge to achieve the necessary clearance of the bed over the legs. One option involves flaring the knee out slightly, operating the microscope pedal with the outside of the foot (Figure 4.10). This lowers the leg significantly and allows the foot to work the pedal with very little elevation of the knee and therefore little disturbance of the surgical bed.

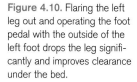

Figure 4.10. Flaring the left leg out and operating the foot pedal with the outside of the left foot drops the leg significantly and improves clearance under the bed.

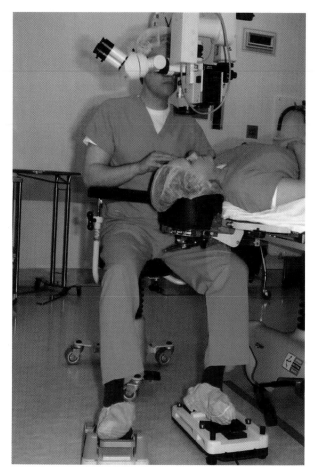

STABILIZING THE HANDS

The greatest advantage of the operating microscope creates the biggest surgical challenge. The high magnification provides excellent visualization of fine tissues and delicate maneuvers, but it exaggerates any aberrant hand movement. Learning to properly stabilize the hands and thereby decrease hand tremor is one of the greatest challenges facing the resident surgeon. It is a vicious cycle. Understandable nervousness from the surgeon causes some tremor, which when viewed under the microscope appears much greater than it actually is. This in turn fosters more nervousness, with even greater tremor, and so on. Keeping the hands well stabilized dramatically increases your comfort level.

Stabilizing the hands involves four steps:

1. The large arm and shoulder muscles must be stable enough to be quiet and nearly motionless throughout the case; they should not really participate.

2. The hands should be stabilized, usually at the wrist.
3. The small hand muscles must be kept loose and relaxed while working.
4. Any tremor may be dampened with counter touch from the nondominant hand.

Stabilizing the Large Arm and Shoulder Muscles

Stabilizing the hands begins by removing the large muscles from the surgical equation. Two important signs indicate that the large muscles are being used: elevation of the shoulders and elevation of the elbows. Lifting the shoulders, as in a "shrug," tightens the muscles all the way down the arms and increases tremor. An erect torso posture drives the shoulders down into a relaxed position (Figure 4.11). If, on the other hand, the surgeon has the chair too high, he

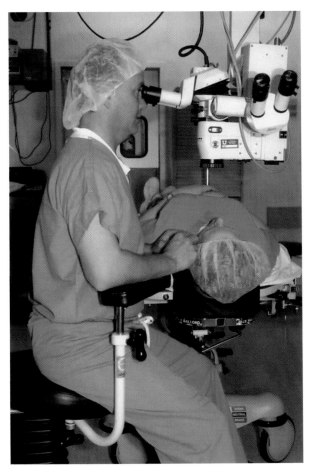

Figure 4.11. Sitting with an erect torso posture lowers the shoulders into a comfortable position. This helps to relax the large shoulder and arm muscles.

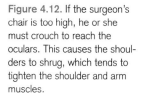
Figure 4.12. If the surgeon's chair is too high, he or she must crouch to reach the oculars. This causes the shoulders to shrug, which tends to tighten the shoulder and arm muscles.

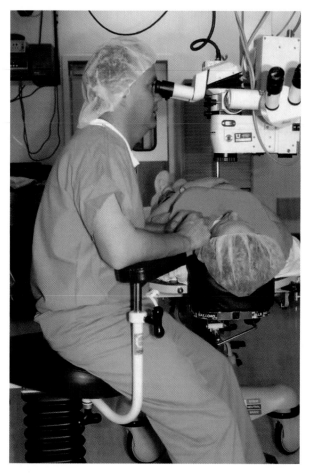

or she must crouch to position at the microscope oculars (Figure 4.12). This position is much more conducive to shrugging the shoulders, causing arm and hand tightness. If you begin to feel tense during surgery, try consciously "dropping the shoulders." This creates a relaxed position with a profound effect on hand stability.

Raised elbows are another sign that the large muscles are too active. This position also elevates the wrists off their support, which greatly destabilizes the hands. There are two ways to ensure that the elbows are staying low and in a relaxed position: The first involves use of a surgical chair that has arm rests (Figure 4.13). This allows excellent support for the entire forearm, from the elbow to the wrist, with the elbow in constant contact with the arm rest. If the surgeon becomes aware that the elbow is not in contact with the arm rest, he or she knows that the elbows are raised and should be dropped into a better position.

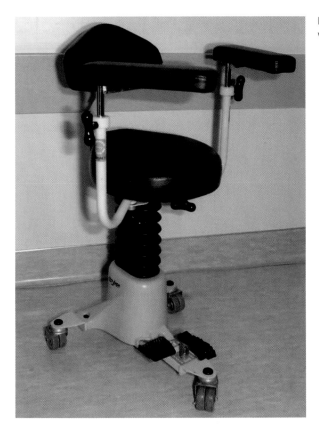

Figure 4.13. Surgical chair with adjustable arm rests.

A second method is use of a wrist rest. Again, elevation of the elbows lifts the wrists off the rest and, on recognizing this, the surgeon should drop the elbows and shoulders if necessary and reposition the wrists back onto the rest.

Stabilizing the Hands at the Wrists

It is critical that the hands be stable at the wrists. A chair with arm rests provides excellent stabilization of the forearm and wrist. Often the arm rests are sufficient and no separate wrist rest is needed, but a wrist rest can also be used separately. This will also help to quiet the arms and shoulders. It is important to understand that the wrist rest (and/or arm rests) needs to be set at different heights depending on the surgeon's position. When working at the 12:00 position, the surgeon's hands have to come over the brow and then "down" to the eye. The wrist support must therefore be set high enough to accomplish this (Figure 4.14). Conversely, when operating temporally, the wrist support can be

Figure 4.14. At the 12:00 position, the wrist rest is set a little higher to allow the hands to come over the brow and "down" to the eye.

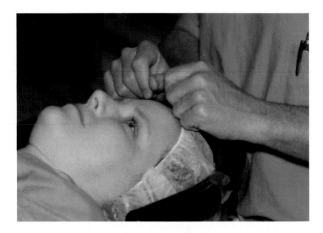

Figure 4.15. At the temporal position, the wrist rest is set lower and the hands come "up" to the eye.

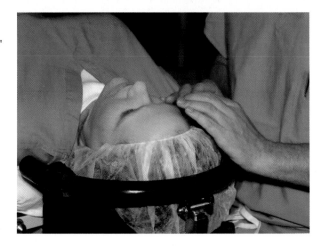

set lower. The surgeon should have the mental image of the wrists set low and the hands coming "up" to the eye (Figure 4.15).

Relaxing the Small Hand Muscles

The next step in reducing tremor is to relax the small hand muscles and keep them tension free. This is extremely difficult without first quieting the large muscles and supporting the wrists. The enemy of such relaxation is a tight grip on the instruments. The beginning cataract surgeon sometimes grips the phacoemulsification hand piece like a vice. It is impossible to reduce tremor with such a grip. Hold the instrument like a pencil and with a light grip (Figure 4.16). This allows the hand to relax. A good practice maneuver is to take a large diameter pen, grip it normally with the thumb and first two fingers of the

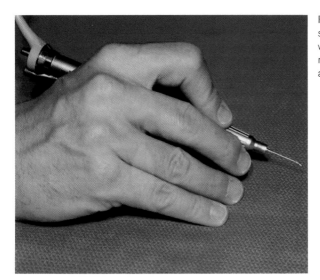

Figure 4.16. The instrument should be held like a pencil with a light grip. This helps to relax the muscles in the hand and reduce tremor.

dominant hand, and practice rotating the pen back and forth as gently as possible. Keep the rest of the hand still, and only move the thumb and two fingers in a gentle rotating motion. This mimics the required maneuvers of cataract surgery, in particular the irrigation and aspiration step during cortical removal, and teaches the surgeon to keep the hands relaxed.

Dampening Tremor With Counter Touch

One of the most effective means of reducing hand tremor is to touch the instrument with the nondominant hand. For example, if a surgeon is holding an instrument in his or her dominant right hand, using the left index finger to just touch the instrument greatly reduces tremor. This obviously is not possible when both hands are being used, but during one-handed maneuvers, the technique is very important and effective. The classic example is during the capsulorrhexis step of cataract surgery, which is a one-handed maneuver usually involving forceps. Grasp the forceps lightly, like a pencil, with the thumb and first two fingers of the dominant hand. Next, take the index finger of the nondominant hand and touch the forceps just below the fingers of the dominant hand (Figure 4.17). This is a very stable hand position and can dramatically reduce hand tremor.

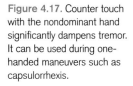

Figure 4.17. Counter touch with the nondominant hand significantly dampens tremor. It can be used during one-handed maneuvers such as capsulorrhexis.

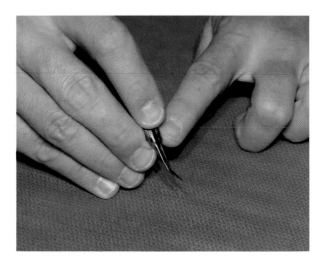

Pearls and Pitfalls of Hand Stabilization

Incorrect hand position causes a few common microscope problems. The first is the tendency for the operative eye to move away from the surgeon during the case, making it difficult to keep the eye centered in the surgical field through the microscope. As discussed previously, this problem can occur if the patient is having trouble fixating on the microscope light or if the patient has rolled her head away from the surgeon. However, by far the most common cause is poor hand position, specifically lifting the hands.

Incorrect hand position, particularly hand lifting, causes several problems, especially during cataract surgery. First, lifting the hands causes the phacoemulsification hand piece to angle downward in the eye. This creates a downward vector during lens sculpting, which is not desirable for zonule preservation. Second, the downward angle of the instrument opens the incision. This allows fluid to escape the eye too quickly, allowing the anterior chamber to shallow, thus increasing the risk of breaking the posterior capsule. Third and most important in the context of the microscope, hand lifting persistently pushes the operative eye away from the surgeon, either down toward the lower lid if the surgeon is at the 12:00 position or toward the nose if the surgeon is operating temporally. This requires more and more adjustment of the microscope position. Beginning surgeons learn to recognize this problem when they are repeatedly using the foot pedal joystick to move the microscope away from them. The remedy is to drop the hands, bringing the wrists and hands back into contact with the wrist rest or arm rest.

Another common microscope problem caused by poor hand position is excessive side-to-side eye movement. This can happen at either the 12:00 or temporal position. The most common cause is failure to keep the surgical instrument centered in the incision. This is one of the most difficult concepts for the new surgeon. The natural tendency is to move the instrument laterally in the incision. Eventually, the end of the incision is reached and at that point the whole eye moves in that direction. The proper technique is to keep the instrument centered in the incision and pivot around that point, like a fulcrum. A good visual concept is to picture the instrument like the oar of a boat. At the wound entrance into the eye, the instrument is locked into place, like the oar-lock on the side of the boat. At this point the instrument (or oar) cannot move laterally, it can only pivot. Learning this technique for intraocular surgery, especially cataract surgery, is essential if the eye is to remain centered in the microscope field. This technique also reduces corneal striae, which improves visualization and safety especially when performing capsulorrhexis.

MICROSCOPE FUNCTION

Once the patient is well positioned, the surgeon is comfortable, and the hands are stabilized, attention is directed to the microscope itself. Four key points in the proper operation of the microscope include

1. Gross maneuvering of the microscope and centering of its axes
2. Positioning and setting the oculars
3. Adjusting the microscope during the case
4. Controlling the lighting

Gross Maneuvering of the Microscope

Modern microscopes can be either ceiling- or floor-mounted. Ceiling-mounted microscopes are useful when there is a dedicated operating room for micro-surgery. They pose less of a physical obstacle within the operating room and do not have to be repositioned with each new patient. Nevertheless, floor-mounted microscopes are equally effective. When the surgeon is positioned at the 12:00 position, the floor-mounted microscope is usually placed on the side of the surgeon's nondominant hand. This allows the surgical instruments to be at the ready for the surgeon's dominant hand. Alternatively, the microscope may always be placed on one side or the other regardless of the operated eye, and it functions very well in this manner. For the temporal approach, the microscope is typically positioned opposite the surgical eye. For example, when operating on a right eye from the temporal approach, the microscope is brought in from the patient's left. Floor-mounted microscopes provide a great advantage in that they can be moved from room to room. Ceiling- and floor-mounted microscopes share most other technical features.

The microscope head is placed on an elaborate swinging positioning arm (Figure 4.18). The various pivot points in the arm can be changed to allow great flexibility in positioning the head of the microscope. Each break point has a tightening mechanism so that the arm can be fixed at that position if desired. The optimal adjustment of the positioning arm is unique for every surgical room and patient orientation. Another important control on the microscope arm, the counterweight setting, determines the vertical excursion of the microscope head when it is positioned and released. This control should be set so that the microscope head remains in place when released.

The centering button, located on the microscope head, centers it in the x-y axes and should be depressed at the beginning of each surgery, thus giving

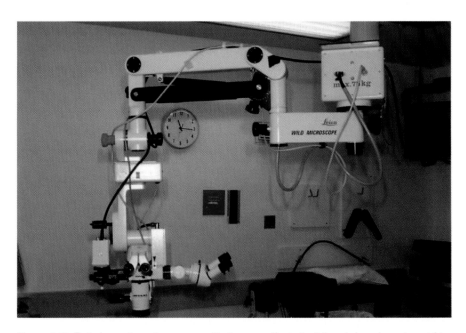

Figure 4.18. Typical operating microscope positioning arm with pivot point controls and counterweight control.

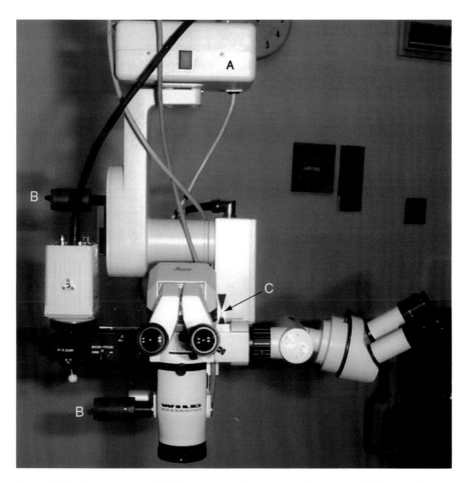

Figure 4.19. Microscope head with (A) a centering button to center the x-y axes, (B) the scale to center the up and down axis, and (C) the positioning handles.

the microscope full excursion in all directions at the start of the case (Figure 4.19A). The head of the microscope is also equipped with large positioning handles. There are two or three handles, usually one on either side of the oculars and often a third on the positioning arm (Figure 4.19B). Typically, handles are fitted with slide-on covers that can be sterilized. A final important initial adjustment, accomplished via the foot pedal, is the centering of the microscope focus in the up and down axis. Most often a scale on the side of the microscope head shows the midpoint of the focus (Figure 4.19C). The microscope may be placed in the middle of the focus axis to slightly above center. Since during surgery, most of the focusing is downward, sufficient excursion in this direction must be available at the start of the case.

Positioning and Setting the Oculars

The three important parameters to be set for the microscope oculars are the pupil distance (PD), the diopter setting, and the tilt. The PD is set either with a small knob on the side of the oculars or simply by manually spreading the oculars to the proper distance. If more than one surgeon will use the microscope during a case or during the course of a day, it may be necessary to adjust the PD intraoperatively under sterile conditions. This is accomplished either with a sterilizeable cap over the adjusting knob, or with sterile covers over the oculars themselves.

The oculars can be set to a specific diopter setting to match the refractive error of the surgeon; most oculars have a range of +/– 5.00 diopters, and each can be set independently to accommodate anisometropia. Alternatively, the surgeon may set the oculars at zero and wear spectacles; this is a good option at teaching institutions where two surgeons may need to view through the primary microscope oculars during the same case.

The oculars also may be tilted vertically. The main use of the vertical tilt is to allow the surgeon to assume the upright torso posture discussed earlier.

Reviewing the Sequence of Setup Steps

To review, the sequence of important steps at the start of the typical case is as follows:

1. Both the patient and surgeon are properly and comfortably positioned.
2. The surgeon checks that his or her feet are on the pedals, the hands are stabilized, and posture is correct.
3. The circulating nurse swings the microscope into position, having first pushed the x-y centering button.
4. The oculars are set.
5. The surgeon then grasps the sterile handles of the microscope, positions the microscope over the surgical eye with low light intensity, and achieves gross focus by manually adjusting the microscope up or down. The microscope focus scale is checked to ensure that the focus is at the midpoint or slightly above.
6. The surgeon then uses the foot pedal to achieve fine focus in the up and down axis. The foot pedal is then used to set the desired magnification level, and again to adjust the fine focus.

With some experience, the entire sequence can be completed in a very short time, and the surgeon is ready to start the case.

Maneuvering the Microscope

Proper use of the foot pedal is the key to efficient and smooth use of the microscope.

Most surgeons find that they cannot feel the microscope pedal well enough with shoes. Many elect to wear shoes that can be easily kicked off, placing surgical shoe covers over their socks, and operating the pedals with their stocking feet. Removing the shoes also lets the knee ride a little lower which helps in clearing the underside of the surgical table.

Most pedals consist of the same basic elements: a joystick to maneuver the scope in the x-y axes, a tab to control the fine focus, and a tab to control the magnification or zoom (Figure 4.20). Some pedals also offer a switch to turn the illumination on and off. Recently designed foot pedals even give some variable control of the illumination.

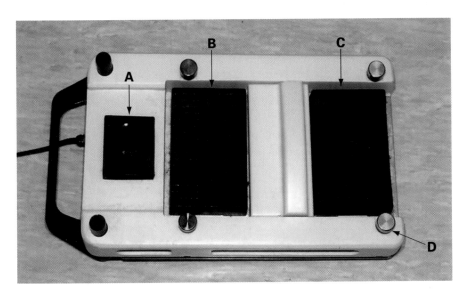

Figure 4.20. Typical microscope foot pedal with (A) x-y joystick, (B) the fine focus tab, (C) the magnification (zoom) tab, and (D) the illumination on/off switch.

An efficient surgery, if properly set up and executed, requires little maneuvering of the microscope with the joystick, because the eye remains well-centered within the microscope's field of view. In fact, technique may be measured to some degree by how little the instrument needs to be adjusted during a case. However, there will inevitably be some maneuvering required, and always some focus and magnification changes during the case, so it is essential that the beginning surgeon learn to smoothly operate the microscope foot pedal.

As mentioned earlier, the foot pedal is usually positioned so that the joystick is away from the surgeon, placing the tabs for the focus and zoom under his or her foot. A recommended position involves the surgeon's heel on the magnification tab and the ball of the foot on the focus tab. In this position, each can be controlled with little foot movement, a toe-down position controlling the focus, and a heel-down position controlling the zoom. Slightly extending the leg and manipulating the joystick either with the side of the toes or the ball of the foot controls the joystick. Experience will allow all of these movements with little or no movement of the surgical field or change in hand position. It is recommended that the surgeon always use the same foot, either right or left, to control the microscope pedal, irrespective of the eye undergoing surgery.

Pearls and Pitfalls of Maneuvering the Microscope

The resident surgeon has the tendency to accommodate through the microscope. This can be fatiguing for the new surgeon, and it hinders the senior mentor's ability to maintain focus while looking through the assistant scope, which typically does not have independent focusing. In the initial setup, it is helpful to focus up with the fine adjustment tab on the foot pedal until the field is just out of focus, and then focus down just until the image comes into focus. This fogging and refocusing limits accommodation through the scope. Since the effect of accommodation is more apparent at high magnification, this maneuver should be performed at high magnification.

Staying in proper focus is also very important. It is common for the beginning surgeon to alter the focus inadequately. This hesitancy usually relates to a lack of comfort with foot pedal manipulation. For example, the surgeon may maintain good focus on the surface of the lens during the initial sculpting step of cataract surgery, but fail to focus down into the lens substance when sculpting more deeply. The focus should concentrate on the point of action. Specifically, the phaco tip must be kept in focus. When coming up into the anterior chamber to remove an air bubble, focus must be adjusted upward, and on moving the instrument down to crack the nucleus, focus is readjusted downward.

Maintaining the proper focus during a typical intraocular case requires multiple adjustments with the focusing tab. If the foot is kept on the microscope foot pedal throughout the entire case, it is easier to make the many small focusing adjustments required.

The level of magnification depends on surgeon preference. Lower magnification allows a wider field of view and greater depth of focus, but it may not offer maximum visualization. High magnification, on the other hand, provides excellent tissue visualization, but reduces the field of view. Maintaining precise focus is also more demanding at higher magnification. The modern microscope offers such easily adjustable magnification that different levels may be used during the same case. For instance, dissection of the scleral flap during a trabeculectomy might best be performed under high magnification since tissue visualization is paramount. Suturing the conjunctival flap in the same case might be done with low magnification since a wider field of view might be advantageous during this step. Excessive magnification changes, however, are usually not necessary and can be fatiguing for the surgeon and particularly for the assistant viewing through the side arm.

Finally, control of the microscope light intensity not only helps reduce the risk of retinal phototoxicity, but also helps to ensure patient cooperation throughout the case. It is not necessary to increase the microscope light to the maximal level to perform good surgery.

For topical cataract surgery, the intensity can be set very low to start. One approach involves turning the microscope light completely off, then nudging the dial up until the light just comes back on, using this intensity as the initial lighting level. All steps up to hydrodissection, including capsulorrhexis, can be performed at this low lighting level. Once hydrodissection is complete, the patient is less photophobic, and the intensity can be turned up, but not much more is needed. For other anterior segment procedures, such as trabeculectomy, the light intensity can be kept low throughout the entire case. It is helpful to mark the light intensity dial on the microscope control panel to help operating room personnel adjust the microscope light.

SURGICAL LOUPES

Surgical loupes provide one great advantage over the surgical microscope. With loupes, the surgeon has the flexibility to view the surgical field rapidly from several angles and positions. For example, many oculoplastic and strabismus surgeries require the surgeon to operate from different positions during the same case. These procedures are particularly amenable to surgical loupes, and in the oculoplastics and pediatric ophthalmic disciplines, loupes are commonly used. Proper use of surgical loupes requires understanding of the principles of magnification, working distance, and field of view.

Magnification

Surgical loupes provide magnification typically ranging from 2 × to 6 ×. Unlike the surgical microscope, the magnification is fixed. The surgeon must decide on what power of loupes to use based on the intricacy of the surgery to be performed. For most ophthalmic procedures, magnification of at least 2.5 × is required; some surgeons recommend at least 3.5 ×. Higher magnification, however, reduces the field of view, and equally important, the depth of field. For example, a 2 × loupe may have a depth of field of 4 inches whereas a 6 × loupe may have a depth of field less than 1.5 inches. Higher magnification loupes require the surgeon to keep the head very still in order to maintain focus, because even slight head movement can translate into a blurred image.

Working Distance

The working distance is also set and not adjustable once the loupes are made. It is important therefore to make sure that this variable is correct. Many factors determine the proper working distance for surgeons, including height and simply where they like to work with their hands. At lower magnification levels, 2.5 × and less, manufacturers typically offer a few different working distances, ranging from about 10 to 20 inches. At higher magnification levels, 3.5 × and higher, the demands of the optics do not allow such flexibility and often the manufacturer offers only one working distance.

Field of View

The field of view varies with the magnification level. The field of view can also be changed optically at the same magnification level. For example, manufacturers can provide different fields of view at the 2 × magnification level, ranging from around 4 inches to 10 inches. Again, however, at the higher magnification levels, the field of view is usually set. The working distance also affects the field of view. A shorter working distance tends to have a smaller field of view.

Pearls and Pitfalls of Surgical Loupes

The most important lesson to learn while working with surgical loupes is to maintain a constant working distance. It is certainly possible to look away from the surgical field over the loupes, but while performing a particular surgical maneuver, it is important to keep the head still to maintain proper focus. When asking for a surgical instrument, the surgeon should keep his or her eyes focused on the tissues and let the scrub nurse hand over the instrument. Although this is not possible in every instance, it should be common practice.

As with surgery through the microscope, good lighting is essential for surgery performed with loupes. Overhead surgical lights provide good illumination and can be easily adjusted by operating room personnel. Many surgeons who use loupes prefer to wear a headlamp, which provides bright and even illumination and is always centered on the desired area. It can be particularly helpful when operating within the orbit or nasal cavity.

KEY POINTS

→ Proper patient positioning includes stabilizing the head neither chin-up nor chin-down in the head rest, ensuring that the eye is parallel to the floor and centered in the microscopic field, and supporting the back and legs in a comfortable position.

→ Proper surgeon positioning includes ensuring freedom of movement of the legs under the operating table, comfortable access to the microscope foot pedal, and a posture allowing for stabilization of the shoulders and hands.

→ The surgeon must be familiar with gross maneuvering of the microscope and centering of its axes; positioning and setting the oculars; adjusting the microscope during the case; and controlling the lighting.

→ With surgical loupes, the surgeon has the flexibility to view the surgical field rapidly from several angles and positions; knowledge of magnification, field of view, and working distance are critical.

SELF-ASSESSMENT TEST

1. Proper patient positioning for the operating microscope includes
   a. The corneal surface should be parallel to the floor
   b. The chin-up and chin-down positions should be avoided
   c. The patient's head is fully onto the head rest
   d. All of the above
2. Common pitfalls in surgeon positioning include (list all that apply)
   a. Surgeon too far away from patient (legs not sufficiently under the table)
   b. Table too high
   c. Shoulders and elbows too low
   d. Pedals poorly positioned
3. Correct setup of the operating microscope includes (list all that apply)
   a. Oculars set
   b. The x-y control decentered toward head
   c. Microscope manually positioned and grossly focused
   d. Fine-focus set in down-focused position
   e. Foot pedal used for fine-focus
   f. Foot pedal used to set magnification
4. The following are true of surgical loupes (list all that apply)
   a. They provide increased mobility for the surgeon requiring magnification.
   b. Higher magnification loupes also provide increased depth of focus and working distance.
   c. Head movement during surgery increases depth perception with loupes.
   d. A headlight may be worn with loupes to improve focal lighting of the surgical field.

For preferred responses to these questions, see pages 223–224.

SUGGESTED READING

Technical manual for the surgeon's specific microscope.

Chapter 5

Surgical Instruments and Blades

Jay M. Lustbader, MD

One of the most important aspects of becoming a proficient ophthalmic surgeon is gaining an understanding of the use of the many instruments and blades ophthalmologists employ. Although the number of surgical instruments can initially be quite daunting, being able to identify and use surgical instruments and blades properly is an essential skill. This chapter introduces you to the major categories of instruments and blades.

The choice of instruments is quite individualized, and in time each surgeon develops a favorite tool for performing a given task. A variety of ways exist for performing the same procedure, and the best way is the one that allows a particular surgeon to accomplish the task with minimal trauma to the tissues. Although detailed discussion of surgical instrumentation and machinery is beyond the scope of this book, equipment company representatives and other experienced surgeons are valuable sources of information in this area. (Most photographs in this chapter are courtesy of Wilson Ophthalmic Corporation; Figure 5.23 is courtesy of Katena Products, Inc.)

SURGICAL INSTRUMENTS

Retractors

Retractors are used to help open the eyelids, both in the office and the operating room.

Figure 5.1. Desmarres lid retractor. Often used when the lids cannot otherwise be opened (eg, lid edema) or in double everting of the lid to look for foreign bodies.

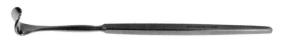

Figure 5.2. Jaffe wire retractor. Used in ruptured globe surgery to avoid applying undue pressure to the globe. Attached to the surgical drapes with a rubber band.

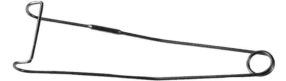

Figure 5.3. Jaeger lid plate.

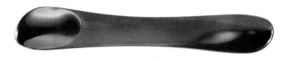

Speculums

Speculums are used to hold the eyelids apart, in order to have better access to the eyeball during a surgical procedure.

Figure 5.4. Barraquer wire. Commonly used in many anterior segment procedures.

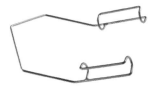

Figure 5.5. Kratz-Barraquer speculum with open blades to allow easy insertion and removal of the phacoemulsification handpiece.

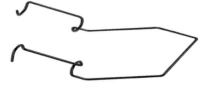

Figure 5.6. Varieties of screw-type speculums, which can be adjusted to the dimensions of the lid fissure as needed. (A) Cook. (B) Lancaster. (C) Williams.

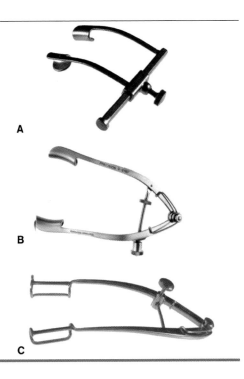

Chalazion Instruments

Clamp and curette are the primary tools used in excising chalazions. The individual shape and size chosen will vary with the size and location of the chalazion.

Figure 5.7. Examples of chalazion eyelid clamp. The clamp is used to hold the lid and provide some hemostasis around the chalazion. Such clamps include variations in cross action, dimensions, and sizes and shapes of the upper and lower "plates."

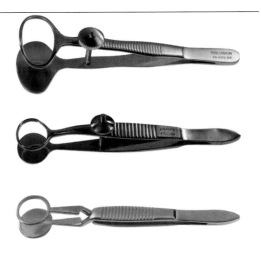

Figure 5.8. Curette used to scoop out the contents of the chalazion; available in sizes of 0 (1.5 mm) to 4 (3.5 mm).

Lacrimal Instruments

This group of instruments is used to locate and clear obstructions of the tear duct. Lacrimal sets may group a dilator to enlarge the punctum, a syringe, and a blunt cannula to introduce solution into the duct, and a lacrimal probe to clear the duct.

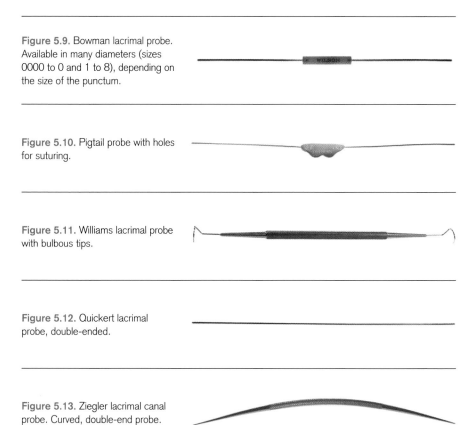

Figure 5.9. Bowman lacrimal probe. Available in many diameters (sizes 0000 to 0 and 1 to 8), depending on the size of the punctum.

Figure 5.10. Pigtail probe with holes for suturing.

Figure 5.11. Williams lacrimal probe with bulbous tips.

Figure 5.12. Quickert lacrimal probe, double-ended.

Figure 5.13. Ziegler lacrimal canal probe. Curved, double-end probe.

Figure 5.14. Ruedemann lacrimal dilator. Dilators are available in a variety of sizes and tips to accommodate the large variety in shapes and sizes of the lacrimal system. The example shown here, designed for use with an infant, has a smooth, round handle and a short taper.

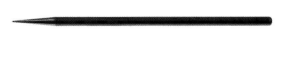

Scissors

A variety of scissors are available for use in ocular surgery. Depending on the surgical purpose, scissors may be blunt or sharp, curved or straight, and may feature either spring or direct action.

Figure 5.15. Stevens tenotomy scissors.

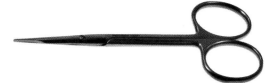

Figure 5.16. Westcott tenotomy scissors with blunt or sharp tips. All-purpose ophthalmic surgery scissors.

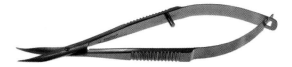

Figure 5.17. Westcott conjunctival scissors. Smaller than tenotomy scissors, also with blunt or sharp tips.

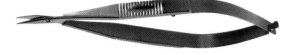

Figure 5.18. Suture scissors are available in many styles. (A) Fine, straight stitch scissors. (B) Jaffe. (C) Needle point. (D) Westcott. (E) Westcott type with wide, serrated handle.

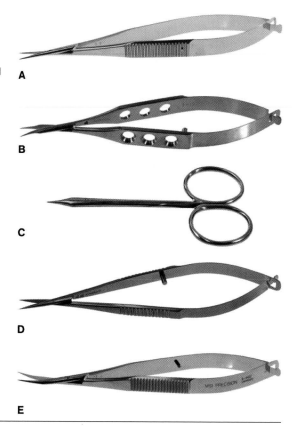

A

B

C

D

E

Figure 5.19. Vannas scissors with sharp pointed tips, available curved or straight. Commonly used scissors for cutting sutures, iris, or fine tissues.

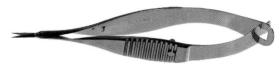

Figure 5.20. Katzin corneal transplant scissors, miniature model, lower blade 12 mm, upper blade with left, strong curve. Corneal scissors are more curved than corneoscleral scissors. Corneal scissors are used to cut the corneal button in corneal transplant surgery. Also designed for cutting to the left or right.

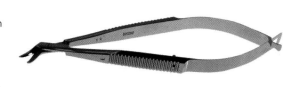

Figure 5.21. Enucleation scissors. Specially designed to reach to the posterior globe to cut the optic nerve during enucleation. This example shows a medium curve; strong and light curves are also available.

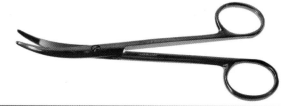

Forceps

Forceps are used for grasping tissues or sutures. Teeth or serrations in forceps help the surgeon grasp ocular tissues to allow suturing, fixation, or dissection. A broad, flat, nontoothed tip aids the surgeon in tying sutures. Some instruments may contain a locking device in the handle.

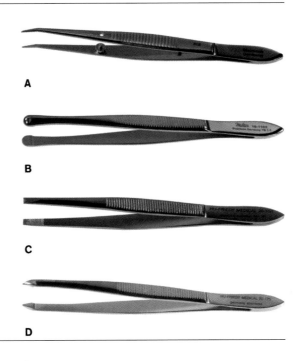

Figure 5.22. Cilia forceps for removal of aberrant cilia. Available in different angle and types of jaws. The examples shown here have a wide, blunted tip to aid in grouping the cilia. (A) Barraquer. (B) Beer. (C) Douglas. (D) Ziegler.

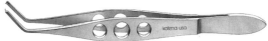

Figure 5.23. Superior rectus forceps are used to grasp the rectus muscles for placement of traction sutures.

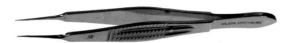

Figure 5.24. Castroviejo suturing forceps, toothed. Available with a tying platform for suture tying. The 0.12 mm (".12") forceps are widely used in a variety of ophthalmic surgeries. They are excellent for grasping and holding fine tissues. The 0.3 mm and 0.5 mm forceps are used when a larger grasp of tissues is needed than is possible with a 0.12 mm.

Figure 5.25. Colibri corneal forceps. A 0.12 mm forceps with a curved handle and tying platform.

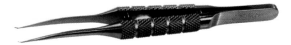

Figure 5.26. Bishop-Harmon forceps. Criss-cross serrated tips. Smaller version of the standard 0.12 mm forceps. Also good for grasping tissue.

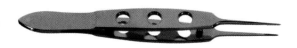

Figure 5.27. Bonn iris forceps. Without teeth, with serrated tips. Smaller version of the standard 0.12 mm forceps, also good for grasping tissue.

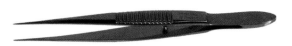

Figure 5.28. Jeweler's forceps. Sharp, fine-tipped forceps available in a variety of designs and sizes, beyond the examples shown here. Often used for suture removal. (A) Straight, strong points. (B) A variation in width and thickness. (C) Curved with fine points. (D) Simple, short, stubby with medium points.

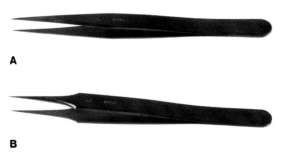

A

B

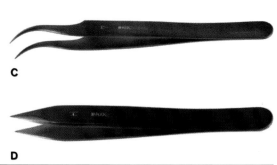

C

D

Figure 5.29. McPherson tying forceps. Many styles of tying forceps are available, including straight and angled designs. Some surgeons prefer to tie sutures with one of each.

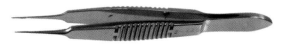

Figure 5.30. Tennant tying forceps. Another example of tying forceps. Round handle with guide pins and platform, for 9/0 to 11/0 sutures.

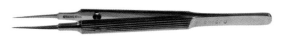

Figure 5.31. Kelman-McPherson angled tying forceps. Angled tying forceps are most commonly used for intraocular manipulations (for example, placing the superior haptic with intraocular lens insertion). They are also useful for grasping intraocular tissues.

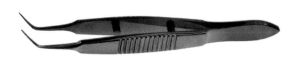

Figure 5.32. Capsulorrhexis forceps. Used to grasp the anterior capsule flap to create the circular curvilinear capsulorrhexis in cataract surgery. The tips can be sharp, cupped, or blunt. This Kraff Utrata example shows a three-hole handle and delicate tips.

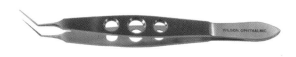

Hooks

Hooks are curved tools used for holding, lifting, or pulling on tissue and intraocular lenses.

Figure 5.33. Sinskey hook. A small hook used in a variety of applications, including IOL positioning, tissue displacement, corneal marking, and many others. The Sinskey hook can be straight or angled.

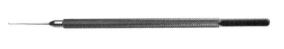

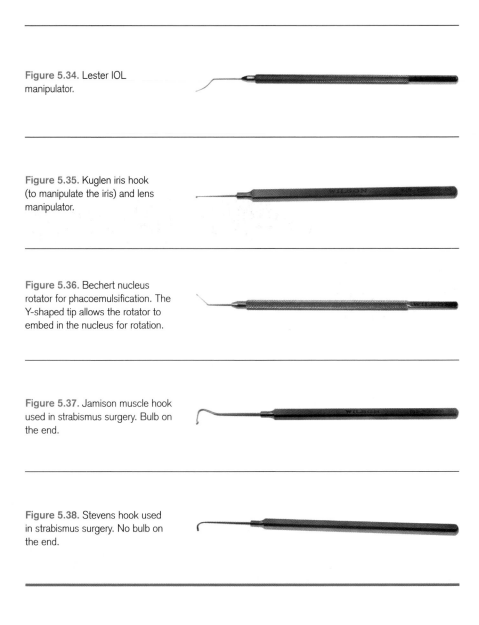

Figure 5.34. Lester IOL manipulator.

Figure 5.35. Kuglen iris hook (to manipulate the iris) and lens manipulator.

Figure 5.36. Bechert nucleus rotator for phacoemulsification. The Y-shaped tip allows the rotator to embed in the nucleus for rotation.

Figure 5.37. Jamison muscle hook used in strabismus surgery. Bulb on the end.

Figure 5.38. Stevens hook used in strabismus surgery. No bulb on the end.

Spatulas

Spatulas are useful in a variety of applications in ophthalmic surgery. They allow gentle, controlled manipulation of tissue.

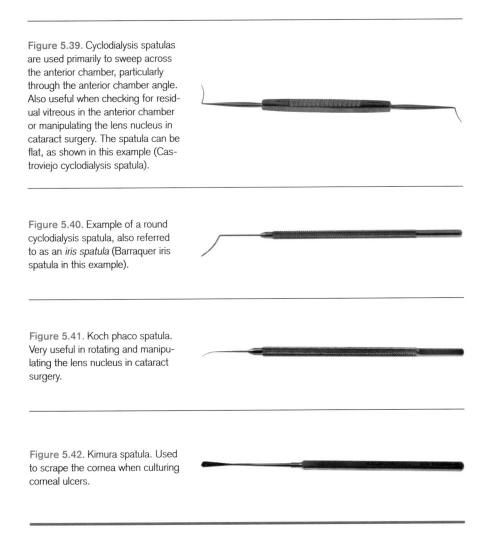

Figure 5.39. Cyclodialysis spatulas are used primarily to sweep across the anterior chamber, particularly through the anterior chamber angle. Also useful when checking for residual vitreous in the anterior chamber or manipulating the lens nucleus in cataract surgery. The spatula can be flat, as shown in this example (Castroviejo cyclodialysis spatula).

Figure 5.40. Example of a round cyclodialysis spatula, also referred to as an *iris spatula* (Barraquer iris spatula in this example).

Figure 5.41. Koch phaco spatula. Very useful in rotating and manipulating the lens nucleus in cataract surgery.

Figure 5.42. Kimura spatula. Used to scrape the cornea when culturing corneal ulcers.

Needle Holders

Needle holders are used to hold the suture needle, which provides the surgeon with more control of the suturing process. In use, the needle holder is cradled like a pencil.

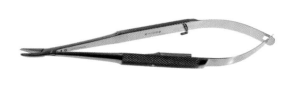

Figure 5.43. Needle holders for suturing can be straight or curved. Additionally, they can be supplied with or without a lock, to hold the needle in place in the jaws. The example shown here is a curved Barraquer needle holder.

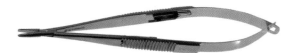

Figure 5.44. Example of a straight needle holder with straight, standard jaws and lock (Castroviejo).

Cannulas

Cannulas are small, tube-like instruments frequently used in ophthalmic surgery to inject or extract fluid or air.

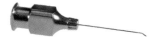

Figure 5.45. Anterior chamber irrigating cannula. Example of Knolle irrigating cannula with 45° angled tip, available in different gauges.

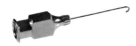

Figure 5.46. J-shaped hydrodissection cannula. Hydrodissection cannulae are available with a variety of tip designs, allowing improved access under the anterior capsular edge.

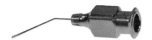

Figure 5.47. Example of a flat-shaped hydrodissection cannula (Seeley).

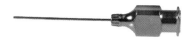

Figure 5.48. Lacrimal cannula. Used to irrigate through the lacrimal system. Available in various gauges and styles of opening. This example is 23 gauge with a front opening.

Other Surgical Instruments

Examples of other specialized instruments used in ophthalmic surgery include punches, calipers, trephines, lens loops, nucleus choppers, and posterior capsule polishers and scrapers.

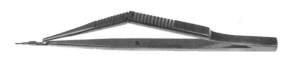

Figure 5.49. Kelly Descemet's membrane punch with serrated squeeze action handle. Used to excise portions of trabecular meshwork during trabeculectomy.

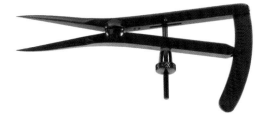

Figure 5.50. Castroviejo caliper. Used in a variety of surgical procedures to measure distances on the eye. This example measures 0 to 20 mm in 1-mm increments.

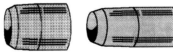

Figure 5.51. Corneal trephines. Blades are used to excise the donor cornea and diseased patient cornea during corneal transplantation.

Figure 5.52. Standard lens loop. Lens loops are used to help in removal of the nucleus in extracapsular cataract extraction.

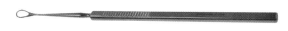

Figure 5.53. Sheets irrigating vectus (another example of a lens loop). Allows irrigation of fluid into the anterior chamber during nucleus extraction.

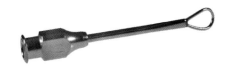

Figure 5.54. Standard phaco chopper. Nucleus choppers are available in many angles (45°, 60°, 90°) and designs. Used in phaco-chop cataract surgery to break the lens nucleus into small pieces.

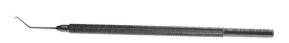

Figure 5.55. Posterior capsule polishers and scrapers come in many designs. Used to remove residual material from the posterior capsule prior to intraocular lens insertion in cataract surgery.

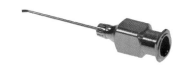

Figure 5.56. Jensen posterior capsule polisher.

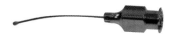

SURGICAL BLADES

Surgical blades are supplied presterilized and are disposable. They either can be supplied preloaded on a handle or inserted into a standard surgical scalpel handle.

Standard Surgical Scalpel Blades

Figure 5.57. Blades for standard surgical scalpels are available in various sizes and shapes (#10 to #15, #20 to #23). Numbers 10 and 15 tend to be the most commonly used in ophthalmology. (A) Rib-back carbon steel. (B) Stainless steel.

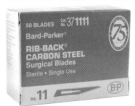

A

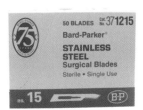

B

Stab Knife Blades

Figure 5.58. A stab knife is used for controlled entry to the anterior chamber for paracentesis and other purposes. A variety of blades and angles are available, including 15° ("supersharp"), 22.5°, 30° and 45°).

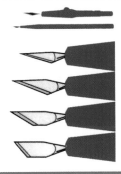

Cataract Surgery Blades

Figure 5.59. Crescent blade. Used for tunneling through the sclera into clear cornea. Straight or angled design.

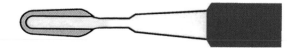

Figure 5.60. Keratome (phaco slit knife). A variety of blade diameters are available (2.5 to 5.2 mm) dependent on the desired incision size for the phacoemulsification procedure. Sharp-tip keratome blades penetrate the cornea easily and provide an optimal fit for the phaco tip. Blunt-tip keratomes (shown) are used to enlarge the phaco incision for intraocular lens insertion. This keratome follows the slit blade incision and the cutting edge creates a precise opening for lens insertion.

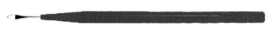

Scleral Blades

Figure 5.61. Blade #57. Also called a "hockey stick blade" due to its unique shape. Often used for creating scleral flaps.

Figure 5.62. Blade #64. This blade has both a straight edge and a rounded edge. In addition to creating scleral incisions, also used for scraping the corneal epithelium.

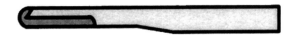

Figure 5.63. Blade #69. The blade is curved all the way around. Useful for creating extracapsular cataract incisions, as well as corneal scraping.

Figure 5.64. Blade #66. Available angled or straight. Used to create lamellar dissections of sclera or cornea.

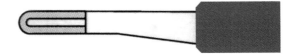

Figure 5.65. Blade #59. Also called a *Ziegler knife*. Used to make a precise entry into the anterior chamber through the limbus.

Figure 5.66. Blade MVR. Also called a *needle knife*. A sharp, diamond-shaped, pointed blade, usually 19 or 20 gauge. Used in vitreous surgery to create the sclerotomies.

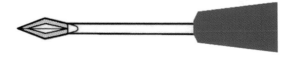

Clear Cornea Blades

Figure 5.67. A variety of widths and angles are available. Can be made of steel or diamond. Frequently with depth markings to ease the creation of clear cornea incisions.

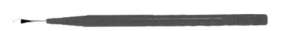

KEY POINTS

→ Scissors for microscopic use have specific design characteristics for the type and direction of incision and tissue involved for dissection. Depending on the surgical purpose, scissors may be blunt or sharp, or curved or straight, and may feature either spring or direct action.

→ Forceps are used for tissue stabilization and suture tying; they vary in size and tip characteristics depending upon desired function. Teeth or serrations in forceps help grasp ocular tissues. A broad, flat, nontoothed tip aids the surgeon in tying sutures. Some instruments may contain a locking device in the handle.

→ Surgical blades vary in size and shape according to tissue dissection and type of incision. They include designs for stab incision, curvilinear incision, and dissection of deep tissue layers.

SELF-ASSESSMENT QUESTIONS

1. Match scissor type with use (list all correct matches):
   a. Vannas: suture cutting
   b. Corneoscleral: cataract wound
   c. Westcott tenotomy: microscopic tenotomy
   d. Stevens tenotomy: microscopic tenotomy
2. Match forceps type with use (list all correct matches):
   a. Castroviejo 0.12 mm forceps, toothed: corneoscleral tissue
   b. Castroviejo 0.12 mm forceps, toothed: fine suture tying
   c. Jeweler's forceps: suture removal
   d. Kelman-McPherson forceps: intraocular lens manipulation
   e. Colibri 0.12 mm forceps: corneal tranplantation
3. Match instrument with use (list all correct matches):
   a. Kuglen hook: iris manipulation
   b. Cyclodialysis spatula: sweep anterior chamber
   c. Lens loop: cataract extraction
   d. Corneal trephine: excise corneal tissue
4. Match blade with use (list all correct matches):
   a. Keratome: phacoemulsification
   b. Scleral blade # 57: scleral flap creation
   c. Scleral blade # 69: extracapsular cataract incisions
   d. Stab knife ("supersharp blade"): anterior chamber entry

For preferred responses to these questions, see pages 223–224.

Chapter 6

Suture Materials and Needles

Jennifer Lee, MD
Keith D. Carter, MD

Surgical techniques for reapproximation of skin edges and support of wounds vary widely; the broad array of suture material allows ophthalmic surgeons individual preferences in ocular surgery. This chapter introduces the characteristics of suture and needle construction that the beginning surgeon must understand in order to minimize tissue damage and maximize wound support. (Chapter 12 reviews the mechanics of proper knot tying and suturing.)

CHARACTERISTICS OF SUTURES

An ideal suture should have ease of handling, correct tensile strength, minimal tissue reactivity, and minimal promotion of bacterial infection. The surgeon must select a suture material with the characteristics that are most appropriate for the cutaneous or ocular wound.

The following definitions are helpful in understanding characteristics of sutures.

> → *Suture-size nomenclature:* A number followed by a dash and a zero describes suture size. In ophthalmology, you will probably use sutures between 2-0 and 10-0. A smaller number indicates a larger suture. The size of the suture affects the tensile strength.
> → *Handling:* The ease of manipulating and tying a suture.

→ *Coefficient of friction:* The force required to move two sliding surfaces over each other, divided by the force holding them together. It is reduced once the motion has started.

→ *Tensile strength:* The amount of force required to break a suture divided by its cross-sectional area. It is a specific feature of the suture composition itself. Strength of the suture also depends on its size; for example, a 6-0 suture is typically more resistant to breakage than a 10-0 suture.

→ *Tissue reactivity:* The amount of inflammatory response evoked by the presence of suture material.

CLASSIFICATION OF SUTURES

Sutures may be classified by the kind of material from which they are made (natural, synthetic, metallic), their internal structure (monofilament vs multifilament), whether or not they are absorbable, and their diameter.

Material

Suture may be composed of natural fibers (silk or gut), synthetic material (nylon, polyglycolic acid, polypropylene), or stainless steel. Selection of suture material involves consideration of absorbability, tensile strength, and handling needs for the situation. No suture is ideal from all standpoints; therefore, the choice of suture material remains the surgeon's preference.

Internal Structure

Monofilament sutures are made of a single strand of material, while multifilament sutures involve braided strands of single filaments. Monofilament suture causes less scarring and tissue reaction. It is easier to remove and has less tissue drag. With monofilament sutures, you need to use a 3-1-1 tying sequence for throws (a *throw* is the tying down of one or more loops; see Chapter 12 for techniques of wound closure). The number of throws you need to use also depends on the memory of the material. Polypropylene (Prolene) is very resilient to being deformed and sometimes requires a 3-1-1-1 sequence as opposed to nylon that may be tied with a 2-1-1 sequence. Braided suture is easier to manipulate, has higher tensile strength, and maintains tension on a wound after the first throw. With braided sutures, you can use a 2-1-1 or 1-1-1 sequence.

Silk sutures are braided and are considered the easiest to handle and tie because the suture deforms exceptionally well.

Absorbability

Absorbable sutures degrade by an enzymatic process or hydrolysis by tissue fluid, occurring from 5 days to 3 months. Common absorbable sutures include gut, chromic gut (treated with a chromic salt to increase its resistance to absorption), synthetic polyester (Biosyn), polyglactin (Vicryl), and polyglycolic acid (Dexon). Absorbable sutures cannot be used where extended approximation of tissue is required. These sutures absorb more quickly in areas of infection and inflammation. They should be used with caution in patients suffering from conditions that may cause delayed wound healing. All absorbable sutures cause a slight foreign body response that causes the gradual loss of tensile strength and suture mass as the enzymatic process dissolves the suture until it is completely gone. This process can cause increased scarring.

Nonabsorbable sutures allow for extended approximation of tissues. Common nonabsorbable sutures include nylon (Surgilon, Monosof, Dermalon), polyester (Ticron, Mersilene), polypropylene (Prolene), silk (Sofsilk), and stainless steel. Nonabsorbable sutures elicit a minimal acute inflammatory reaction that is followed by a gradual encapsulation of the suture by fibrous connective tissue. Some nonabsorbable sutures, such as Prolene, can remain indefinitely in a deep closure. However, they must be removed if used on the skin.

Absorbable Suture Material

There are four types of absorbable suture material: gut/chromic, Vicryl/ Dexon, Polysorb, and PDS II/ Biosyn. Table 6.1 summarizes each category.

Gut suture is composed of strands of collagenous material prepared from the submucosal layer of the small intestine of healthy sheep or from the seromucosal layer of the small intestine of healthy cattle. It is packaged in a solution of isopropanol, water, and triethanolamine. The suture dries out quickly and becomes stiffer and more difficult to handle; therefore, gut should be opened immediately before usage. Chromic gut is treated with chromic salt solution, which allows maintenance of its tensile strength for a longer time. Care should be taken to avoid crushing or crimping this relatively fragile suture material. Gut is useful in situations where tissues need to be approximated for 4 to 8 days. It is not useful in the closure of sites subject to expansion, stretching, or distention unless other sutures are used deeper in the tissue for structural support. This suture should be avoided in patients with sensitivity to collagen or chromium.

Table 6.1. Absorbable Suture

Type	Primary Material	Filament Type	Tensile Strength	Wound Support	Complete Absorption	Comments
Natural						
Gut; gut chromic	Collagen	Mono	Poor at 7–23 days	4–8 days	Variable	Absorbs more rapidly in inflamed or infected tissue
Synthetic						
Vicryl, Dexon	Polyglactin; polyglycolic acid	Multi	75% at 14 days 5% at 30 days	7–10 days	60–90 days	Less tissue reaction than gut
Polysorb	Glycolide/lactide	Multi	70% at 14 days 55% at 21 days	15–20 days	56–70 days	–
PDS II; Biosyn	polydioxanone; polydioxanone/ glycolide/trimeth-ylene carbonate	Mono	70% at 14 days 25% at 42 days	15–20 days	90–110 days	May need additional throws

There are many synthetic absorbable polyester and polyglycolic acid ophthalmic sutures, the most common of which are outlined in Table 6.1 in order of fastest absorption to slowest absorption. Vicryl (polyglactin 910) and Dexon (glycolic acid) are braided sutures with similar absorption properties. They elicit lower tissue reaction than gut suture. These sutures offer wound support for 7 to 10 days. Absorption is complete between 60 and 90 days. Skin sutures may cause localized irritation after 7 days. Polysorb (glycolide/lactide polyester) is a braided suture and offers wound support for 15 to 20 days. Absorption is complete between 56 and 70 days. PDS II (polydioxanone) and Biosyn (glycolide, dioxanone, trimethylene carbonate) are monofilament sutures and are similar in absorption properties. They offer wound support for 15 to 20 days and are completely absorbed by 90 to 110 days. Additional throws may be necessary for these monofilament sutures.

Nonabsorbable Sutures

There are five types of nonabsorbable sutures: silk, Prolene/Surgipro, nylon, Ticron/Mersilene, and stainless steel. Table 6.2 summarizes each category.

Silk suture (Sofsilk, Perma-Hand) is considered the gold standard for handling and is made from natural proteinaceous silk fibers called *fibroin*. The material is derived from the domesticated silkworm species *Bombyx mori*. Silk suture is braided and coated with a wax mixture to reduce capillarity and increase the ease of passage through tissue. Silk sutures are not absorbed, but progressive degradation of the proteinaceous fiber may cause a very gradual loss of the suture's tensile strength over time. This suture enhances bacterial infectivity.

Polypropylene (Surgipro, Prolene) is a monofilament suture with no change in tensile strength over time. This suture resists involvement in infection and has been successfully employed in contaminated and infected wounds to eliminate or minimize later fistula formation and suture extrusion. The lack of adherence to tissue has facilitated the use of polypropylene suture as a pull-out suture. This material does not deform easily and may require extra throws to avoid knot slippage.

Nylon sutures are available in both monofilament (Monosof, Dermalon, Ethilon) and braided (Surgilon, Nurolon) forms. The braided suture is coated with silicone to increase the ease of passage through tissue and to reduce capillarity. This suture is not absorbed, but progressive hydrolysis of the suture may result in gradual loss of tensile strength over time. Nylon has easier handling than polypropylene, but may still require an extra throw with the monofilament version.

Polyester suture composed of polyethylene terephthalate (Ticron, Mersilene) is a braided suture that is not absorbed and does not degrade over time. It has a higher coefficient of friction and maintains tension on a wound after the first throw.

Table 6.2. Nonabsorbable Sutures

Type	Primary Material	Filament Type	Tensile Strength	Degradation	Comments
Natural					
Sofsilk, Perma-Hand	Fibroin	Multi	None in 365 days	Some	Gold standard for handling
Stainless steel	Stainless steel	Mono or multi	Permanent	None	Telecanthus repair
Synthetic					
Prolene, Surgipro	Polypropylene	Mono	Permanent	None	Resists involvement in infection
Nylon (many brands)	Nylon	Mono or multi	20% per year	Some	
Ticron, Mersilene	Polyethylene terephthalate	Multi	Permanent	None	

Stainless steel suture is composed of 316L stainless steel, a type of molybdenum-bearing steel that is more resistant to corrosion than the conventional chromium-nickel stainless. It is available in both monofilament and multifilament forms. It offers extremely high tensile strength and is used for telecanthus repair.

Suture Size

The diameter of sutures may range from thread-like to microscopically thin. The larger the suture, the smaller the number that is assigned to it. Tables 6.3 and 6.4 list the sizes of sutures commonly used for extraocular and intraocular surgery.

Table 6.3. Examples of Sutures for Extraocular Surgery

Suture Size	Type and Use
2-0	2-0 Vicryl: strong stitch to use as deep anchoring sutures on cheek flaps
3-0	3-0 Gore-Tex CV-3: for indirect browplasty 3-0 silk: to loop the rectus muscles in scleral buckle surgery 3-0 Vicryl: strong stitch to use as deep anchoring sutures on cheek flaps or for subcutaneous closure of forehead and scalp
4-0	4-0 silk: reverse cutting needle for traction sutures 4-0 silk: taper needle for bridle sutures under extraocular muscles 4-0 Vicryl: short half-circle reverse cutting needle, especially useful for lateral tarsal strip 4-0 Vicryl: long reverse cutting needle for thicker subcutaneous closure or as an anchoring suture 4-0 chromic: long reverse cutting needle for Quickert suture and suturing oral mucosa 4-0 chromic: short half-circle needle useful for suturing the flaps for external dacryocystorhinostomy
5-0	5-0 nylon: for brow skin closure 5-0 Prolene: blue color especially useful for repair of lacerations in the brow hairs 5-0 Vicryl: for subcutaneous and orbicularis muscle closure 5-0 chromic: for medial spindle operation used double armed 5-0 fast-absorbing gut: used for skin closure 5-0 Dacron: for scleral buckle attachment to the sclera, superior oblique tuck, or posterior fixation sutures in strabismus
6-0	6-0 Vicryl: double armed for tarsal fracture operation and Jones tube anchoring suture 6-0 nylon: for skin closure of eyelid and periocular skin and to intubate and tie stent used with pigtail probe for repair of canalicular lacerations 6-0 fast-absorbing gut: for conjunctival closure
7-0	7-0 Vicryl: suture for closure of conjunctiva and skin

Table 6.4. Examples of Sutures for Intraocular Surgery

Suture Size	Type and Use
4-0	4-0 silk: traction suture that can be passed under muscles and through the lids
5-0	5-0 Vicryl: suture on a spatula needle for strabismus surgery used double armed to pass a locking stitch through the muscles and 1/2 thickness through the sclera
7-0	7-0 Vicryl: suture for traction through the cornea
8-0	8-0 Vicryl: taper-point "BV" needle for the conjunctival wound in a trabeculectomy 8-0 silk: used for scleral closure in open globes
9-0	9-0 Prolene: iridodialysis repair with a straight or large curved needle 9-0 nylon: used for scleral closure near the limbus 9-0 Vicryl: suture on a BV needle for bleb revision or conjunctival defects
10-0	10-0 nylon: closure of cornea and flap of trabeculectomy. Must be a dark color in order to identify the suture for postoperative laser suture lysis 10-0 Prolene: iris or scleral fixation suture of intraocular lens

NEEDLES

Suture needles are classified by two primary characteristics: curvature and shape (Figures 6.1 and 6.2). Shapes include 1/8 circle (45°), 1/4 circle (90°), 3/8 circle (135°), 1/2 circle (180°), 5/8 circle (225°), bi-curve, compound curve, and straight. Different diameters are available, usually selected to match the diameter of the suture material being used. The 3/8 needle is used most commonly. The 1/2 needle is useful in tight spaces. Straight needles are used in the anterior chamber to suture without disturbing the lens.

Points are classified as either taper or cutting. Cutting needles can be conventional cutting, reverse cutting, or spatula. The needle point determines how easily sutures are passed through tissue. Taper points push through tissue. In ophthalmology these needles are usually labeled "BV" for blood vessel repair and are used primarily for delicate tissue (eg, the conjunctiva in a trabeculectomy procedure, in which the seal around each suture pass is essential to prevent leaking). Cutting needles are more commonly used; their cutting action facilitates the needle penetration of tissue. Reverse cutting needles are the most versatile and cut on the outside curve of the needle. Conventional cutting needles cut on the inside curve and can create a bigger hole as the needle tends to move superiorly out of the wound. Spatula needles facilitate lamellar passes

Figure 6.1. Four basic shapes of needle points used in ocular surgery. (A) Taper point. A cone-shaped single point on a round shaft; used for delicate tissues. (B) Cutting. A triangular point with two-sided cutting edges and an upper cutting edge; largely replaced by the reverse-cutting needle. (C) Reverse cutting. A triangular point with two-sided cutting edges and a lower cutting edge; used for resistant tissue. (D). Spatula. A rhomboid-shaped point with two-sided cutting edges; used in the corner and the sclera where the plane of penetration must be precise. (Reprinted, with permission, from Newmark E, *Ophthalmic Medical Assisting: An Independent Study Course,* Fourth Edition, San Francisco: American Academy of Ophthalmology; 2006.)

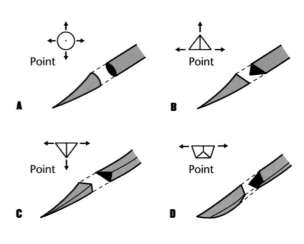

Figure 6.2. Basic shapes of curvature of needles used in ocular surgery. (A) 1/4 circle. (B) 3/8 circle. (C) 5/8 circle. (D) 1/2 circle. (E) Compound curve. (Illustration by Mark M. Miller)

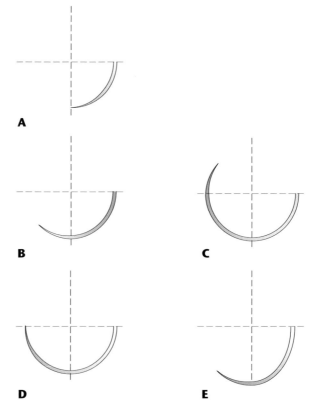

and are commonly used in scleral buckle surgery or strabismus surgery; the flat bottom surface facilitates partial thickness passes through the thin sclera without penetrating the interior scleral wall.

When suturing, always grasp the needle one-third of the way from the suture end in order to avoid damaging the functional integrity of the needle or dulling the cutting surfaces. When handling 7-0 size suture or smaller, always grasp the suture to pull it through the tissue rather than the needle, as you can easily snap the needle off of the end of the suture.

KEY POINTS

→ Suture material is classified by composition, internal structure, absorbability, and size.
→ Common nonabsorbable sutures include silk, nylon, and polypropylene.
→ Common absorbable sutures include gut/chromic, polyglactin 910 (Vicryl)/glycolic acid (Dexon), and glycolide/lactide (Polysorb).
→ Surgical needles are classified by shape, size, and point.

SELF-ASSESSMENT TEST

1. The advantages of monofilament suture include (list all that apply)
   a. Less tissue reaction and scarring
   b. Ease of passage through tissue
   c. Requires fewer throws for stability in knots
   d. Rapidly absorbed
2. The following are nonabsorbable sutures (list all that apply)
   a. Silk
   b. Nylon
   c. Gut
   d. Prolene
   e. Vicryl (polyglactin 910)
3. Vicryl (polyglactin 910) and Dexon (glycolic acid) (list all that apply)
   a. Maintain tissue support for 7 to 10 days
   b. Incite greater tissue reaction than gut suture
   c. Are absorbed in 60 to 90 days
   d. Are monofilament sutures

4. Spatula needles (list all that apply)
  a. Are cutting needles
  b. Are useful for vascular repair
  c. Facilitate lamellar passes in tissue
  d. Are commonly used in scleral buckle surgery or strabismus surgery

For preferred responses to these questions, see pages 223–224.

Part III

Specific Aspects of Surgery

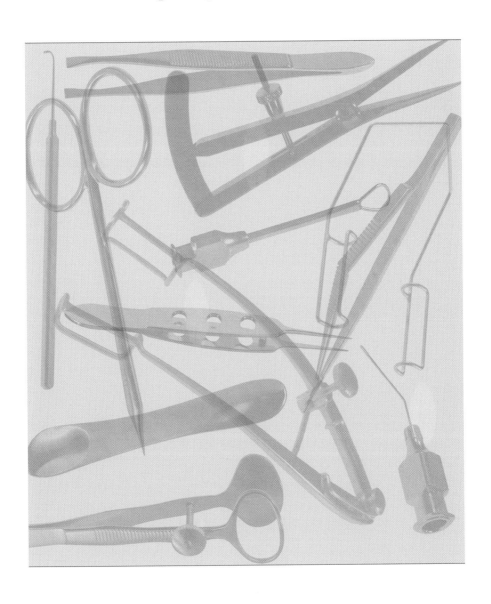

Chapter 7

Patient Safety Issues

Andrew G. Lee, MD

The ophthalmologist-in-training should be cognizant of the specific issues and precautions that are necessary to ensure the safety of the patient during ophthalmic surgery. This chapter discusses four major areas of patient safety in the ophthalmic operating room:

→ Surgery on the incorrect eye
→ Improper intraocular lens insertion
→ Medication errors
→ Iatrogenic fires in the operating room

The American Academy of Ophthalmology (AAO) in conjunction with the American Society of Ophthalmic Registered Nurses (ASORN) has published a series of Patient Safety Bulletins to inform ophthalmologists of systematic practices that can prevent these and other errors from occurring. (See "Suggested Reading" in this chapter for additional information.) The recommendations in this chapter are guidelines for patient safety and should not be construed as a "standard of care." Surgeons, hospitals, or operating rooms may differ in individual approaches, documentation, detail, or scope of their safety protocols and procedures. The content of this chapter is in no way intended to substitute for or replace local institutional policies.

SURGERY ON THE INCORRECT EYE

Surgery on the incorrect eye is the most feared but fortunately preventable medical error in the ophthalmic operating room. Wrong-site surgery is not unique to ophthalmology and is a significant medical, legal, and public relations problem affecting all surgical specialties. The wrong-site error is usually the result of a system or process failure in patient identification, confirmation, or verification of the site of surgery. These types of errors are preventable if the appropriate precautions are taken routinely. From 1985 to 1986, the Physician Insurers Association of America reported 331 closed claims for wrong-site surgery. The Joint Commission on Accreditation of Healthcare Organizations (JCAHO) reported that wrong-site surgery (1995 to 2001) was one of the top ten reported medical errors ($n=152$). Ambulatory care centers were a common location (58%) for this error. Surgery on the wrong eye (eg, enucleation) can be particularly devastating if the fellow unoperated eye still requires surgery despite having had the normal eye removed.

Common causes for wrong-site surgery include poor communication between the surgeon and the patient; inadequate communication among members of the surgical team; reliance upon memory only for the site identification; inadequate preoperative assessment of the patient; or insufficient or inaccurate verification procedures of the operative side. Patients might not identify the surgical site accurately during the informed consent process (eg, patients with language barriers, cognitive impairment, or anxiety over the procedure), in the preoperative area, or during the surgical marking of the site. Surgical team members and ancillary personnel might not properly verify the site of surgery or might over-rely upon the surgeon to make the correct decision. It has been documented that members of the surgical team in some wrong-site cases feared pointing out the error to the operating surgeon. Additional contributory factors in wrong-site surgery have included: involvement of more than one surgeon; performance of multiple procedures on the same patient; time pressure to complete the preoperative procedures more quickly; physical deformity or morbid obesity that might alter the usual set-up of equipment or positioning of the patient; distractions during the identification process; and failure to confirm the site.

In order to prevent wrong-site surgery, the verification process for the operative site should be performed consistently and routinely including:

→ Formal written procedures and protocols for surgical team members to identify and confirm the operative eye. Surgeons should review their individual hospital or operating room protocols periodically.

→ The informed consent form should clearly and explicitly state the operative procedure and the operative eye without the use of potentially confounding abbreviations (eg, OD, OS, IOL).

→ The chart, the preoperative orders for pupil dilation, the regional anesthesia orders, and the surgical prep site should be reviewed by the nurse, anesthetist, resident, fellow, and other surgical team members and all should agree.

→ Verification with the patient (or patient's family if the patient is unable to respond or is a minor) prior to pupillary dilation, anesthesia, surgical prep and drape, or the incision

→ Oral verification of the correct operative site by multiple members of the surgical team

→ Availability of the medical record in the room with explicit written documentation of the operative site

→ Availability and review of the pertinent imaging studies in the operating room

→ Marking of the operative eye (eg, using a marking pen and writing the surgeon's initials at the site)

→ Review of the written verification checklist of all documents referencing the intended operative procedure and site (eg, the medical record, preoperative dilation and surgical preparation orders, the imaging studies and their reports, the informed consent document, the operating room record, the anesthesia record, and direct observation of the marked operative site on the patient)

→ In the case of enucleation, evisceration, or exenteration, the surgeon should perform a final additional verification of the preoperative pathology (eg, intraocular tumor) in the operative eye by direct examination (eg, dilated fundus exam in the operating room)

→ Signature confirmation of completion of the checklist to ensure that all of the above intraoperative steps have been performed

→ A final confirmatory check by the surgeon in the operating room before the incision is made (without relying on memory alone)

INCORRECT INTRAOCULAR LENS PLACEMENT

In addition to wrong-eye surgery, ophthalmic surgeons must prevent errors related to intraocular lens (IOL) placement after cataract extraction. IOL errors may relate to power, size, or type of lens. These errors may lead to a suboptimal postoperative corrected acuity, may require additional optical correction, or may require additional surgery (eg, IOL exchange). In one series of 700 medico-legal cases in ophthalmology, 154 (22%) cases were related to cataract extraction. Of these, IOL errors were the primary cause in one-third of claims. In claims from the Ophthalmic Mutual Insurance Company (OMIC) from 1987 to 1997 claims related to cataract surgery were 33% of the total and of these IOL errors were the majority. Numerous errors may contribute to an incorrect IOL insertion:

→ Use of an outdated or inaccurate IOL power calculation formula
→ Use of the incorrect A-constant in IOL power calculation formula
→ Incorrect axial length (biometry) or keratometry measurements for IOL power calculations
→ Transcription or data entry errors into the IOL power calculation program
→ Inappropriate surgeon selection of postoperative refractive target or IOL style
→ Calculation of IOL insertion for the incorrect patient or incorrect eye
→ Insertion by the surgeon of an incorrect IOL for the particular patient (eg, wrong patient, patients with the same or similar name operated on the same day, wrong eye, wrong procedure)
→ Incorrect labeling or packaging of the IOL by the manufacturer or defective IOL

In one study (*n*=154) of cataract surgery IOL-related errors, 54% were due to erroneous axial length measurement, 38% were anterior chamber depth (ACD) estimation errors, and 8% were corneal power measurement errors. Errors in IOL manufacturing, packaging, or labeling represented less than 1% of the total errors. In order to prevent IOL-related errors, the surgeon or appropriate team member should consider the precautions shown in Table 7.1.

MINIMIZING MEDICATION ERRORS: COMMUNICATION ABOUT DRUG ORDERS

Medication errors are preventable events that may threaten patient safety in the operating room. In 1999, the Institute of Medicine of the National Academies reported that 44,000 to 98,000 deaths occur each year in the United States from medical errors; medication errors constitute a significant proportion of these cases. Common medication errors include: incorrect administration (type,

---

Table 7.1. Precautions for IOL Procedures

In order to prevent IOL-related errors, the surgeon or appropriate team member should consider the following precautions:

1. Ensure that technicians are adequately trained in the techniques for biometry and keratometry measurements and perform periodic technician quality control checks.
2. Perform periodic calibrations of the ultrasound A-scan unit and keratometer.
3. Perform measurements (eg, axial lengths, keratometry) in both eyes for comparison (internal control) and to identify outlying values.
4. Repeat measurements in difficult or complex cases (eg, high myopia, asymmetric refraction) to document the reproducibility of the results.
5. Confirm by repeat measurements results that appear unexpectedly high or low.
6. Review preoperative biometry and keratometry results. (surgeon)
7. Maintain a written IOL calculation checklist that contains patient information, keratometry, axial length, and primary and alternate IOL power, style, and size. (surgeon)
8. In the operating room, check actual IOL information directly against the IOL calculation check-list information. (surgeon)
9. Show the IOL label and verbally confirm the IOL model number and power as the lens is passed to the surgeon for implantation. (circulating nurse, scrub nurse, surgical assistant, with confirmation by the surgeon)
10. Perform a final visual inspection of the IOL under the microscope for any lens defects or deposits. (surgeon)

---

dose, or route); inaccurate product labeling, packaging and nomenclature; and inaccurate compounding, dispensing, or distribution.

Like wrong-site surgery, medication errors are a common cause of malpractice claims; in the Physician Insurers Association of America database (n=117,000 claims), medication errors were the second most common cause for a claim. In a review of 700 medico-legal cases in ophthalmology, medication errors were the third most frequent complaint. In data from the Ophthalmic Mutual Insurance Company, claims for medication errors are more costly than the average claim and more likely to result in indemnity payments.

Factors that might contribute to medication errors include:

→ Incomplete, inaccurate, or unreviewed patient information (eg, known allergies, complete list of medications, complete medical history, complete surgical history, laboratory or radiographic results)
→ Incomplete or unavailable drug information (eg, lack of up-to-date warnings, product information, or drug interactions)
→ Use of standing preoperative or postoperative orders without physician review of patient allergies, potential drug interactions, or duplication of medications

→ Use of standing orders to "continue preoperative medications" without physician review of existing medication list for allergies, indications, contraindications, drug interactions, or adverse effects

→ Miscommunication between surgeon and other members of the surgical team (eg, nurse, technician, or pharmacist) regarding drug orders (eg, not hearing the complete order, deleting or inserting a word like "with" or "without" epinephrine from the verbal order)

→ Illegible handwriting, confusing letters (eg, lowercase letter "l" and the number "1", letter "o" for number "0", or letter "z" for number "2"), or incomprehensible verbal order

→ Confusion between drugs with similar sounding or similar written names or packaging. These medications should be identified as "high risk," labeled with both trade and generic names, and should not be stored in close proximity. Some examples of ophthalmic and systemic medications that might be confused and have been reported to the United States Pharmacopeia list include the following (brand names are capitalized):
  - atropine and Akarpine
  - Betagan and Betoptic
  - Betoptic and Betoptic S
  - erythromycin and azithromycin
  - Murocel and Murocoll-2
  - Ocufen and Ocuflox
  - Ocufen and Ocupress
  - Refresh (lubricant eye drops) and ReFresh (breath drops)
  - TobraDex and Tobrex
  - Voltaren and tramadol
  - Voltaren and Ultram

→ Misuse or misinterpretation of zeroes and decimal points in drug dosing

→ Confusion of metric and English system units in dose

→ Use of illegible, inaccurate, or inappropriate abbreviations

→ Inaccurate or inappropriate labeling as a drug is prepared and repackaged into smaller units or into different delivery instruments (eg, syringes mislabeled)

→ Environmental factors (eg, poor lighting, heat, noise and interruptions) that can distract health professionals from their medical tasks

→ Failure to follow institution/facility policies and procedure

→ Presence of medications that may be safe in one route (eg, topical or subconjunctival) but devastating if administered via a different route (eg, intraocular gentamicin causing macular infarction)

Table 7.2. Procedures That Help Minimize Medication Error

---

1. Complete and accurate medication list in the chart
2. Careful review of all relevant patient information by the surgeon (eg, known allergies, complete list of medications, complete medical history, complete surgical history, and laboratory or radiographic results)
3. Avoidance of the use of "standing orders" to "continue preoperative medications" without review of medication list, indications, allergies, and doses
4. Explicit communication between surgeon and other members of the surgical team (eg, nurse, technician, pharmacist) regarding drug orders including "digit by digit" repetition of dose (ie, two-three rather than twenty three).
5. Legible handwriting with block handwriting; avoidance of abbreviations and Latin; complete spelling of drug names, route, and dosage; and avoidance of inappropriate or illegible decimal points in dosage orders
6. Use of leading zero before decimal points (eg, 0.1) and avoidance of use of trailing zero after decimal point (eg, 5. rather than 5.0)
7. Complete adherence to institutional, hospital, and facility policies and procedures regarding labeling of all medications, containers (eg, syringes), and solutions
8. Discarding unlabeled solutions or medications in the operating room
9. "Forcing functions" that eliminate the presence of medications from the surgery table that may be safe in one route but unsafe via a different route (eg, gentamicin, cytotoxic agents, and hypertonic saline)
10. Review of patient allergies prior to administration of drug
11. Individual verbal and written confirmation of medication orders and verification of dose, route, and medicine prior to administration

---

→ Lack of confirmation of medication order and verification of dose, route, and medicine prior to administration of drug

Table 7.2 lists procedures that help minimize the possibility of medication errors.

PREVENTING SURGEON-RELATED FIRE IN THE OPERATING ROOM

Most hospitals and operating rooms have internal policy and procedure manuals regarding fire prevention and safety. The surgeon in training should be familiar with these rules and regulations. The Massachusetts Department of Public Health reviewed incidents of fire in the operating room. They identified three key elements necessary for combustion: an oxidizer, a fuel source, and an ignition source. Although a patient may require oxygen in the operating room, an oxygen-enriched environment is a major factor in many surgical fires. In an oxygen-enriched or nitrous oxide–enriched environment, surface fibers (eg, fabric, body hair, vellus hair) can flash (propagate flames) and then ignite more-combustible fuels at the edge of the initial surface.

The patient's health status should be reviewed carefully and the requirement for oxygen should be documented and confirmed as necessary. Oxygen and nitrous oxide levels can build up under the surgical drapes, and tenting of the operative drape (eg, with a Mayo stand) may allow the oxygen to dissipate and gravitate towards the floor. Oxygen can also build up from leakage around endotracheal tube cuffs.

Ophthalmic surgeons should avoid if possible creating an "oxygen tent" that could allow unnecessary build up of oxygen. A fire can be precipitated by a spark or other ignition source in this highly oxygen-enriched environment. The risk for these fires can be reduced by draping the patient's entire face with nasal cannula oxygen allowing the oxygen to dissipate more rapidly.

Cautery units and lasers may act as an ignition source and are more hazardous with oxygen in use because of the lowered temperature threshold for ignition. These units should be activated only when the tip is in view and should not be allowed to contact drapes or other combustible material. Hot-wire cautery devices (Figure 7.1) should not be set down on or near flammable material (eg, gauze or drapes) while still hot. A safety holster should be employed for all devices with active electrodes and set with the tip away from flammable items. If oxygen must be employed, then the lowest temperature setting for the cautery unit to achieve therapeutic effect should be employed. If possible, the oxygen should be held for at least 1 minute prior to use of the cautery and then restarted after the cautery is completed. Other potential ignition sources in the operating room include electrosurgical units, surgical lasers, fiberoptic light sources, and incandescent or static discharge sparks. Electrosurgical or cautery units should only be activated when the tip is visible and should be deactivated before the tip is removed from the surgeon's view.

Combustible substances that may ignite or act as fuel after a fire in the operating room (Figure 7.2) include the surgical drapes and material (eg, gauze, sponges, adhesive tape, drape, hoods, and gown); surgical equipment (eg, plastic or rubber products, anesthesia masks, and tubes); operating room ointments, solvents, and solutions (eg, degreasers, petrolatum, aerosols, paraffin, wax, alcohol, adhesives, and tincture solutions); and the patient's hair (eg, head hair, eyebrows, mustache, or beard). The hair can be made less flammable by coating with water-soluble lubricating jelly preoperatively. In ophthalmic surgery, the drapes may cover the eyebrows but in other cases the brow is exposed in the surgical field and coating the eyebrows might be of benefit if oxygen will be in use. Volatile solutions (eg, liquid alcohol) should not be allowed to pool in the field, on the patient, or in open containers and sufficient

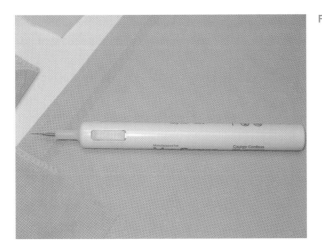

Figure 7.1 Cautery unit.

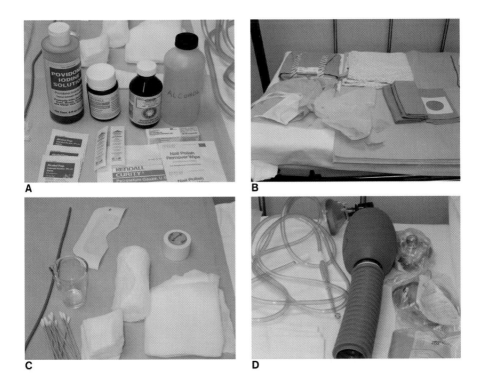

Figure 7.2. Combustible substances that may ignite or act as fuel after a fire in the operating room. (A) Solvents and solutions (eg, alcohol, adhesives, tincture solutions). (B) Surgical drapes, patient's cap and gown. (C) Dressings (gauze, sponges, adhesive tape). (D) Surgical tubing.

time should be allowed for drying of any topically applied solutions (eg, adhesives, tinctures, surgical prep solutions, and ointments). Alcohol-based surgical preps may contribute to fires if the vapors are trapped by the drapes and come into contact with a heat source. Patients should be advised preoperatively against the use on the day of surgery of skin, facial, and hair care products or medications that may contain potential combustible substances (eg, alcohol-based solutions). This includes skin care creams, moisturizers, hair tonics, conditioners, and topical ointments).

KEY POINTS

→ Steps to avoiding wrong eye surgery include formal written protocols for preoperative confirmation of correct eye, avoidance of abbreviations for proposed operated eye in the consent form, surgeon use of marking pen to identify correct eye in the operating room, and final verification of correct eye pathology by direct surgeon's examination.

→ Incorrect IOL insertion may be caused by faulty power calculations, data transcription errors, surgeon judgment errors, and manufacturer labeling errors.

→ Steps to avoid medication errors include ensuring presence and review of complete and accurate medication list in the chart, avoidance of standing orders and abbreviations, reconfirmation of dosage digit by digit between surgeon and medical team members, and eliminating potentially unsafe medications from the surgical suite.

→ Causes of operating room fires include oxygen-enriched environment (under surgical drape), contact of cautery unit with flammables, excess flammable solutions such as cosmetics, and volatile operating room solutions.

SELF-ASSESSMENT TEST

1. Procedures to prevent wrong-eye surgery include (list all that apply)
   a. Formal written procedures and protocols for surgical team members to identify and confirm the operative eye
   b. Informed consent form that clearly and explicitly states the operative procedure and the operative eye without the use of potentially confounding abbreviations

    c. Availability of the medical record in the room with explicit written documentation of the operative site

    d. Marking of the operative eye (eg, using a marking pen and writing the surgeon's initials at the site)

2. Factors in incorrect IOL insertion include (list all that apply)

    a. Incorrect perimetry data

    b. Incorrect axial length (biometry) or keratometry measurements for IOL power calculations

    c. Calculation of IOL insertion for incorrect patient or incorrect eye

    d. Incorrect optical coherence tomography measurement of macular thickness

3. Common sources of medication error include (list all that apply)

    a. Use of standing preoperative or postoperative orders without physician review of patient allergies, potential drug interactions, or duplication of medications

    b. Miscommunication between surgeon and other members of the surgical team (eg, nurse, technician, and pharmacist) regarding drug orders

    c. Patient self-medication in the operating room

    d. Illegible handwriting, confusing letters, or incomprehensible verbal order

    e. Confusion between drugs with similar sounding or similar written names or packaging

4. Combustible substances that may ignite in the operating room include (list all that apply)

    a. Surgical drapes and material

    b. Anesthesia masks and tubes

    c. Operating room ointments, solvents and solutions

    d. The patient's hair

For preferred responses to these questions, see pages 223–224.

SUGGESTED READING

American Academy of Orthopaedic Surgeons and American Association of Orthopaedic Surgeons. *Wrong-Site Surgery* [Advisory Statement]. October 1997.

American Academy of Orthopaedic Surgeons. *Report of the Task Force on Wrong-Site Surgery.* September 1997, revised February 1998. Available at: www.aaos.org; accessed 1/15/2006.

Brandt RW. Daily safety for you and your patient. *AORN J.* 1972;16:64–67.

Brick DC. Risk management lessons from a review of 168 cataract surgery claims. *Surv Ophthalmol.* 1999;43:356–360.

Courtright P, Paton K, McCarthy JM, et al. An epidemiologic investigation of unexpected refractive errors following cataract surgery. *Can J Ophthalmol.* 1998;33:210–215.

ECRI. Fire hazard created by misuse of Duraprep solution. *Health Devices.* 1998;28:286.

ECRI. Fires during surgery of the head and neck area. *Health Devices.* 1979;9:50–52.

ECRI. Fires from oxygen use during head and neck surgery. *Health Devices.* 1995;24:155–157.

ECRI. The patient is on fire! A surgical fires primer. *Health Devices.* 1992;21:19–34.

Eliminating Wrong Site Surgery [Patient Safety Bulletin]. A Joint Statement of the American Academy of Ophthalmology, the American Society of Ophthalmic Registered Nurses (ASORN) and the American Association of Eye and Ear Hospitals. 2001. Available at: www.aao.org/resources; accessed 1/15/2006.

Ellis JH. Faulty A-scan readings present potential liability. ARGUS 1994. From OMIC Publication Archives. Available at: www.omic.com/ resources/risk_man/deskref/clinical/21.cfm; accessed 1/15/2006.

Institute of Medicine. *To Err Is Human: Building a Safer Health System.* Washington, DC: National Academies Press; 2000.

Joint Commission on Accreditation of Healthcare Organizations. *Lessons Learned: Wrong Site Surgery.* Sentinel Event Alert [serial online]. August

28, 1998;6. Followup alert December 5, 2001. Available at: www.jcaho.org; accessed 1/15/2006.

Kohnen S. Postoperative refractive error resulting from incorrectly labeled intraocular lens power. *J Cataract Refract Surg.* 2000;26:777–778.

Massachusetts Department of Public Health. Health care quality safety alert: Preventing operating room fires during surgery. 2002. Available at: www. mass.gov/dph/dhcq/pdfs/orfires.pdf; accessed 1/15/2006.

Medication Errors [Patient Safety Bulletin]. A Joint Statement of the American Academy of Ophthalmology, the American Society of Ophthalmic Registered Nurses and the American Association of Eye and Ear Hospitals; 2002. Available at: www.aao.org/resources.

Minimizing Wrong IOL Placement [Patient Safety Bulletin]. A Joint Statement of the American Academy of Ophthalmology, the American Society of Ophthalmic Registered Nurses and the American Association of Eye and Ear Hospitals; 2005. Available at: www.aao.org/resources.

Morris R. Wrong power IOL inserted during cataract surgery [serial online]. *OMIC Digest.* 2000:11. Available at: www.omic.com/resources/risk_man/ deskref/closedclaim/35.cfm; accessed 1/15/2006.

Murphy EK. Liability for incorrect intraoperative medications. *AORN J.* 1989;50:1106–1108.

National Patient Safety Foundation. *Agenda for Research and Development in Patient Safety.* 2000. Available at: www.npsf.org; accessed 1/15/2006.

Norrby N, Grossman L, Geraghty E, et al. Accuracy in determining intraocular lens dioptric power assessed by interlaboratory tests. *J Cataract Refract Surg.* 1996;22:983–993.

Olsen T, Olesen H. IOL power mislabeling. *Acta Ophthalmol (Copenh).* 1993;71:99–102.

Olsen T. Sources of error in intraocular lens power calculation. *J Cataract Refrac Surg.* 1992;18:125–129.

Smith HE. The incidence of liability claims in ophthalmology as compared with other specialties. *Ophthalmology.* 1990; 97:1376–1378.

Verification and marking of the operative eye. In: *The Johns Hopkins Hospital Wilmer Ophthalmological Institute Interdisciplinary Clinical Practice Manual*, revised August 2000.

Chapter 8

Aseptic Technique and the Sterile Field in the Operating Room

Scott C. Sigler, MD
Ensa K. Pillow, MD

Aseptic and sterile techniques have evolved tremendously since the medical profession in 1879 officially accepted Joseph Lister's antiseptic principles of surgery. Often, the terms are used interchangeably.

Today, much time and care is taken to minimize the possibility of infection resulting from surgical procedures. According to the *Guideline for Prevention of Surgical Site Infection* published by the Centers for Disease Control, the most common pathogens involved in postoperative eye infections are coagulase-negative *Staphylococcus*, *Staphylococcus aureus*, and gram-negative bacilli. This chapter introduces you to the agents, techniques, and practices used to reduce the infection rate following surgical procedures.

SKIN PREPARATION

The most common antiseptic agents used in preoperative preparation of the surgical site are iodophors, alcohols, and chlorhexidine gluconate.

Iodophors, such as povidone-iodine (Betadine), are compounds based on a bactericidal complex of iodine and a nonionic surface-active agent. In ophthalmic surgery, iodophors are the agents used most frequently in prepping the skin around the eyes as well as the conjunctiva. They provide bactericidal effect as long as they are present on the skin, and they are effective against gram-positive and gram-negative bacteria, viruses, fungi, protozoa, and yeasts.

Because they can cause skin irritation, iodophors should be avoided in patients with iodine allergies.

Alcohol (70% to 90% ethyl or isopropyl) works by denaturing proteins. It is effective against gram-positive and gram-negative bacteria, fungi, some viruses, and tuberculosis mycobacteria. Alcohol is readily available, inexpensive, and acts rapidly. Because it is easily ignited and burns rapidly, alcohol must be handled carefully in the operating room (see Chapter 7 for discussion of preventing fire in the operating room).

Chlorhexidine gluconate (Hibiclens), as with iodophors and alcohol, is effective on a broad spectrum of microbial activity including gram-positive and gram-negative bacteria, fungi, and spores but has less activity against viruses and tuberculosis mycobacteria. It works by disrupting the cell membrane of microorganisms. Because residues tend to accumulate on skin with repeated use, chlorhexidine has a long duration of action (~6 hours). Toxicity can occur if the agent comes in contact with the middle ear or the cornea.

APPLICATION OF ANTISEPTIC AGENTS

In practice, if gross contamination is present from dirt, soil, or debris (as may occur in dirty lid lacerations), the skin should first be cleaned by irrigating the site with saline. The application of antiseptic begins with the eyelashes. Cotton swabs are soaked with the antiseptic and applied along upper and lower lash lines. Next, the surgical site is cleaned by applying the antiseptic using gauze sponges in concentric motions starting from the central operative site and moving peripherally. This process is repeated three times with new sponges/ 4×4s for each new application. Avoid moving from peripheral to central site because contamination can occur. All areas that will be exposed during the surgery should be covered with the antiseptic (Figure 8.1). For intraocular surgeries, drops of povidone-iodine 5% are placed on the conjunctiva to reduce the risk of endophthalmitis.

For surgeries requiring local anesthetic, an alcohol swab is used to clean the injection site. Once the local anesthetic is injected, skin preparation begins as described above.

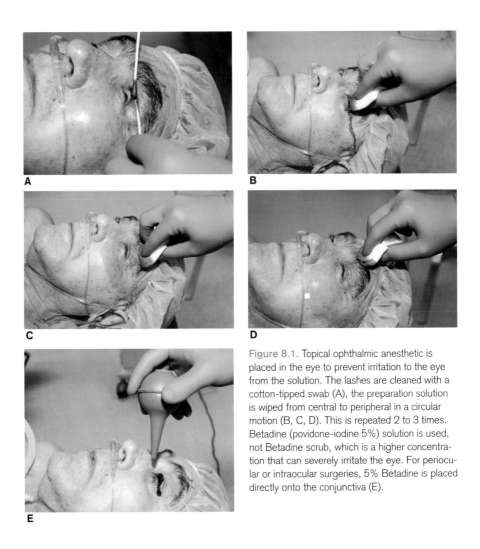

Figure 8.1. Topical ophthalmic anesthetic is placed in the eye to prevent irritation to the eye from the solution. The lashes are cleaned with a cotton-tipped swab (A), the preparation solution is wiped from central to peripheral in a circular motion (B, C, D). This is repeated 2 to 3 times. Betadine (povidone-iodine 5%) solution is used, not Betadine scrub, which is a higher concentration that can severely irritate the eye. For periocular or intraocular surgeries, 5% Betadine is placed directly onto the conjunctiva (E).

HAND SCRUBBING

Scrubbing of the surgeon's hands and forearms involves antiseptic agents similar to those used in preparing the skin of the surgical site. Before hand scrubbing is begun, the surgeon dons a surgical mask and head cover. Any jewelry and artificial nails should be removed. Generally accepted practice for the first scrub of the day includes a total duration of 5 minutes; however, the optimum duration of scrubbing is not proven, with some studies suggesting that 2 minutes is effective. (Also see "Hand Preparation" in Chapter 3.)

Here are the four basic steps in scrubbing the hands and forearms:

1. Begin by cleaning underneath the fingernails and then proceed proximally from the hand to the elbow (Figure 8.2A, B).
2. Elevate the tips of the fingers so the water and scrub solution drain down and off the elbow (Figure 8.3A, B).

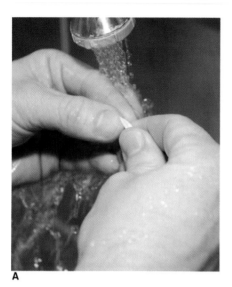
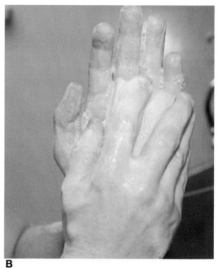

A   **B**

Figure 8.2. Hand scrubbing. (A) The nails are addressed first with solution, water, and the nail pick. (B) Note while scrubbing, the fingertips are pointed up.

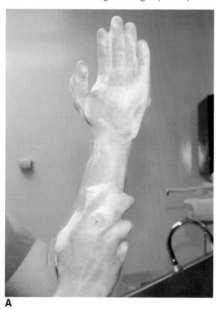
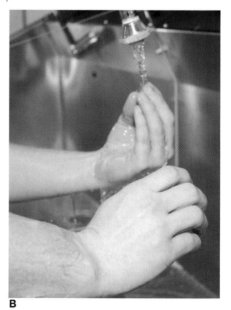

A   **B**

Figure 8.3. Hand scrubbing. (A) The arms are scrubbed after the hands and the movement goes down to the elbows. (B) The hands are rinsed first and followed by the forearms. The fingertips stay pointed up.

3. Following the scrub, keep the hands up and away from the body with elbows bent.
4. When rinsing, take care to avoid allowing runoff to contaminate the opposite hand or forearm.

GOWNING AND GLOVING

Microorganisms are shed from hair, exposed skin, and mucous membranes. Surgical attire including scrubs, caps/hoods, masks, gowns, and gloves are used to minimize the exposure. In most operating rooms, a scrub technician is available for help with gowning and gloving. Informing the scrub tech of your gown and glove size is helpful. In situations where a technician is not available, you should be familiar with the technique of gowning and gloving yourself. This section discusses the procedures for doing so with or without an assistant.

Sterile towels are made available in the operating room for drying, usually placed on top of a gown. After a thorough scrub, the surgeon carefully grasps the towel, extending the arm and hand over the sterile field the least distance possible, without dripping water from the freshly scrubbed hands onto the field (see "Sterile Field" later in this chapter).

The towel is opened up with the right hand underneath the towel. The left hand is dried on the side of the towel opposite the right. Drying starts with the tips of the fingers and goes down to the elbows. Then the towel is flipped onto the left hand so the right hand can be dried on the opposite side. The towel is discarded away from the sterile field into the appropriate bin.

Gown and Glove Procedure With an Assistant

After you have dried your hands and forearms, the technician approaches, holding the gown open with the inside toward you. Insert your hands and arms into the arm holes, but do not extend your hands through the open end of the gown arms. The technician then offers the right glove, typically fingers down. Extend the right hand into the glove as it exits the open end of the gown arm, so that the glove may be pulled onto the hand and over the gown arm with minimal exposure of the hand. The same procedure is then performed with the left glove. The technician or scrub nurse ties the inside back of the gown and you rotate to wrap the outside gown around the back, which is also tied by the technician or scrub nurse.

Gown and Glove Procedure Without an Assistant

The technician typically places the gown on the table with the back facing up. The goal is to touch anywhere within the interior of the gown without touching the outside surface. Carefully grasp the inside of the gown, near the top of the gown. With both hands and gravity, the gown is allowed to unfold and open up. Then carefully slide your hands and arms into the inside arm holes, keeping your hands within the sleeves. The scrub nurse or technician will tie the back of the gown. Figure 8.4 illustrates the steps of putting on sterile gloves without an assistant.

DRAPING

Draping refers to the positioning of sterile drapes around the surgical site to avoid contamination of the incision, instruments, and supplies. Depending on the procedure and the surgeon, draping can vary tremendously. The goal is to drape inside the previous prepped sterile field so that the drapes expose the sterile area to be operated, while covering the nonsterile surrounding areas. It is usually recommended that the edges of the drapes be adhesive material so there is a tight seal that prevents movement of the drapes during the procedure. The draping is performed after the antiseptic solution is used (Figure 8.5).

STERILE FIELD

The sterile field consists of the surgeon's gown in front of the chest to the level of surgical site, hands up to elbows, and of the surface of the draped table. If there is any nonoperative time during the surgery (eg, waiting on proper instruments), hands should remain in the sterile field; they are usually clasped together in front of chest or placed on the operating table. Arms should not be crossed with hands in axilla because the axillary region is considered nonsterile. Hands below the waist are considered no longer sterile. If an instrument falls below the level of the table, it is considered nonsterile and appropriately replaced. A nonsterile member of the surgical team should remove the instrument, not the surgeon or scrub technician. If the surgeon must cough or sneeze during the surgery, the correct technique is to back away from the table and cough or sneeze into the surgical mask. The surgeon should not turn his or her head since masks are not sealed to the face.

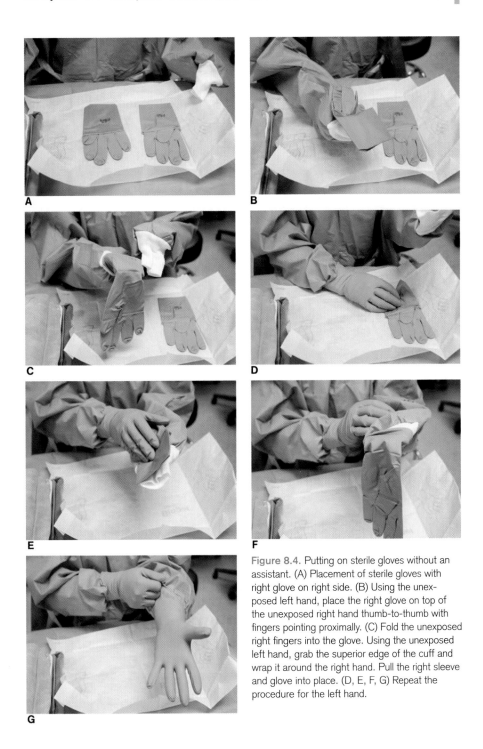

Figure 8.4. Putting on sterile gloves without an assistant. (A) Placement of sterile gloves with right glove on right side. (B) Using the unexposed left hand, place the right glove on top of the unexposed right hand thumb-to-thumb with fingers pointing proximally. (C) Fold the unexposed right fingers into the glove. Using the unexposed left hand, grab the superior edge of the cuff and wrap it around the right hand. Pull the right sleeve and glove into place. (D, E, F, G) Repeat the procedure for the left hand.

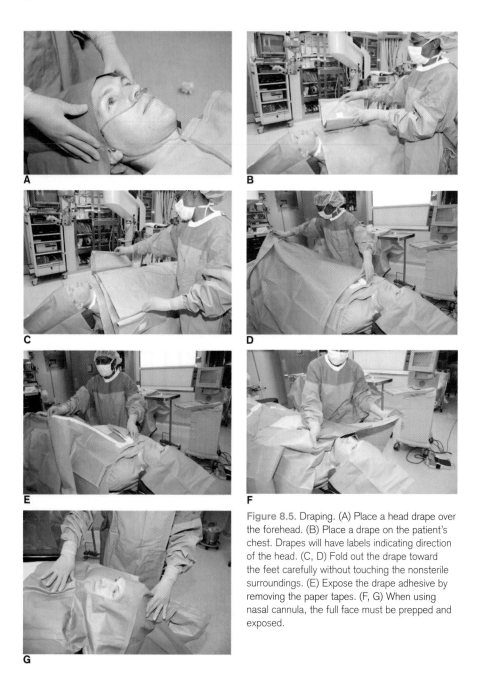

Figure 8.5. Draping. (A) Place a head drape over the forehead. (B) Place a drape on the patient's chest. Drapes will have labels indicating direction of the head. (C, D) Fold out the drape toward the feet carefully without touching the nonsterile surroundings. (E) Expose the drape adhesive by removing the paper tapes. (F, G) When using nasal cannula, the full face must be prepped and exposed.

When using a surgical microscope, move the instrument by the sterile handles; there are areas that are within reach that may not be sterile. If there is any question as to what is sterile or not within the field, it is best to ask before touching. If there is a question during the procedure whether an unsterile object touched an area, instrument, or part of the surgeon's gown or gloves, stop the procedure and cover the suspected area with a sterile towel. If the surgeon's arm is contaminated, a sterile sleeve can be placed over it. A contaminated glove should be replaced.

When passing another gowned person, the persons should pass face-to-face or back-to-back. The surgeon should never walk by the sterile field with his or her back to the sterile drapes or to the sterile surgical table.

KEY POINTS

→ The most commonly used skin preparation agents include iodophors, such as povidone-iodine (Betadine), alcohols, and chlorhexidine gluconate.

→ The steps involved in the surgical hand scrub include cleaning the fingernails first, then scrubbing proximally from the hand to the elbow, elevating the tips of the fingers so the water and scrub solution drain down and off the elbow.

→ Gowning and gloving involves maintaining the sterility of the outer (surgical field) surfaces, touching only the inner surfaces while donning.

→ The sterile field consists of the surgeon's gown in front of chest to the level of surgical site, hands up to elbows, and surface of the draped table.

SELF-ASSESSMENT TEST

1. Povidone-iodine (list all that apply)
   a. Is bacteriostatic
   b. Is effective against gram-positive and gram-negative bacteria
   c. Is ineffective against fungi and yeast
   d. Only rarely induces an allergic reaction
   e. Is less effective than alcohol for antisepsis

2. The surgical hand scrub (list all that apply)
   a. Is proven to require 5 minutes minimum
   b. Proceeds from hand proximally to elbow
   c. Always begins with the surgeon's dominant hand
   d. Must include cleaning the fingernails
   e. All of the above

3. In the gown and glove procedure without an assistant (list all that apply)
   a. The surgeon exposes the hands through the end of the gown arms
   b. The surgeon grasps only the inside surface of the gown
   c. The surgeon must tie the back of the gown
   d. Gloves are donned before the gown
   e. All of the above

4. The sterile field typically includes (list all that apply)
   a. The area between the surgeon's waist and shoulders
   b. The microscope base
   c. The surgical field
   d. The underside of the operating table, if above the waist
   e. All of the above

5. In intraocular surgeries, the current accepted practice to reduce the rate of endophthalmitis is
   a. Preoperative lash trimming
   b. Preoperative saline irrigation
   c. Preoperative topical antibiotics
   d. Preoperative povidone-iodine

For preferred responses to these questions, see pages 223–224.

SUGGESTED READING

Brunicardi CF, Andersen DK, Billiar TR, et al. *Schwartz's Principles of Surgery.* 8th ed. New York: McGraw-Hill; 2004.

Buzard K, Liapis S. Prevention of endophthalmitis. *J Cataract Refract Surg.* 2004;30:1953–1959.

Ciulla TA, Starr MB, Masket S. Bacterial endophthalmitis prophylaxis for cataract surgery: an evidence-based update. *Ophthalmology.* 2002;109:13–26.

Mangram AJ, Horan TC, Pearson ML, et al. Guideline for prevention of surgical site infection, 1999. Centers for Disease Control and Prevention (CDC) Hospital Infection Control Practices Advisory Committee. *Infect Control Hosp Epidemiol.* 1999;20:250–278.

Phillips N. *Berry and Kohn's Operating Room Technique.* 10th ed. St. Louis: Mosby; 2003.

Phippen MI, Wells MP. *Patient Care During Operative and Invasive Procedures.* Philadelphia: WB Saunders; 2000.

Speaker MG, Menikoff JA. Prophylaxis of endophthalmitis with topical povidone-iodine. *Ophthalmology.* 1991;98:1769–1775.

Chapter 9

Ophthalmic Anesthesia

Steven J. Gedde, MD
Yunhee Lee, MD, MPH

Adequate ophthalmic anesthesia is required for safe ocular surgery; it may be attained through local (topical, intraocular, regional) or general administration. Anesthesia techniques have evolved in recent years along with surgical procedures. Many intraocular surgeons utilize regional anesthesia by an orbital block, although topical anesthesia is growing in popularity, especially in small-incision cataract surgery. General anesthesia is typically reserved for patients who are not candidates for regional or topical anesthesia. This chapter reviews the anesthetic agents in common use, techniques of ocular anesthesia, appropriate patient selection, and possible anesthesia complications.

SEDATION

The goal of sedation is to achieve anxiolysis (minimal sedation), amnesia, or somnolence. The choice of sedative agents depends on three factors:

1. The patient: Frequently, patients undergoing ophthalmic surgery are elderly and may have multiple systemic illnesses that need to be considered.
2. The procedure: Surgical procedures differ in complexity, length, and degree of patient discomfort. Patients undergoing longer procedures may benefit from continuous sedation in order to tolerate lying quietly for a prolonged period.

3. The surgeon: Some surgeons prefer that the patient be awake and cooperative, especially when topical anesthesia is used.

The desired level of sedation may be achieved with the intravenous administration of rapid-onset, short-duration drugs. For example, the benzodiazepine
midazolam (Versed) can be titrated in 0.5 to 1.0 mg increments to a total dose
of 2.0 mg. Alternatively, the barbiturate methohexital (Brevital) or the seda-
tive-hypnotic propofol (Diprivan) may be given in 15 to 20 mg increments to
a total dose of 30 to 60 mg. The advantages of methohexital and propofol are
rapid onset (45 to 90 seconds) and short duration (5 to 15 minutes) of sedation, compared with an onset of 3 minutes and duration of 1 to 3 hours for
midazolam.

Patient safety always comes first. Oversedation or increased drug sensitivity may lead to hypoventilation, hypoxia, obstructed breathing, and disorienta-
tion. Oxygen and an Ambu bag for manual ventilation should always be readily available when sedation is given. Sedation must be attained while providing
cardiopulmonary stability, good operating conditions, and a rapid return to
the patient's preoperative mental and general physical status. Most ophthalmic
surgery is performed on an outpatient basis, so a rapid return to full recovery
is extremely important. In many cases, sedation is administered by anesthesia
personnel who have experience with the medications and can focus solely on
their management during the surgical procedure. (Also see "Minimizing Medication Errors: Communication About Drug Orders" in Chapter 7.)

LOCAL ANESTHETIC AGENTS

Local anesthetic agents may be delivered topically, intraocularly, or by orbital
injection. It is important to be familiar with the onset and duration of action
of the various agents, as the expected length of the surgical procedure influences the choice of agent. Local anesthetics administered by orbital injection
are frequently combined to produce a rapid onset and long duration. Certain
adjuvant drugs are also commonly used to augment their effect.

Topical Anesthetic Agents

Table 9.1 lists topical anesthetic agents in common use for ocular surgery. The
onset of anesthesia following instillation of each of the commonly used agents
is within 15 to 20 seconds and lasts 15 to 20 minutes. Superficial punctate kera-

Table 9.1. Topical Anesthetic Agents

Generic Name	Trade Name	Concentration (%)	Duration of Action (min)
Cocaine		1–4	20
Proparacaine	AK-Taine Alcaine Ophthaine Ophthetic	0.5	15
Tetracaine	Ak-T-Caine Pontocaine Anethaine	0.5	15
Lidocaine	Xylocaine	2–4	15

topathy may result from all of the topical anesthetic agents due to epithelial toxicity and inhibition of epithelial cell division.

Cocaine

Cocaine was one of the first anesthetic agents used in ocular surgery. In addition to its anesthetic effect, cocaine is unique in that it produces vasoconstriction. Cocaine's use for topical anesthesia in ocular surgery has largely been abandoned because it produces corneal clouding due to epithelial toxicity. Its most common current use is for surface anesthesia of the upper respiratory tract in select oculoplastics procedures.

Proparacaine

Proparacaine 0.5% produces a rapid onset of corneal and conjunctival anesthesia with the least amount of discomfort. A single drop is adequate to anesthetize the eye for applanation tonometry. However, 1 drop should be administered every 5 minutes for approximately 5 doses to produce deeper anesthesia for ocular surgery.

Tetracaine

Tetracaine 0.5% has a slower time of onset and invokes more discomfort than proparacaine. The deeper anesthesia it produces still makes it a very useful agent in ophthalmic procedures. Local vasodilation results from its direct action on blood vessels.

Lidocaine

Lidocaine 4% solution or 2% gel is often used topically in ophthalmology. Of all anesthetic agents for ocular use, it is the least toxic to the corneal epithelium. Topical lidocaine produces deep anesthesia with a relatively long duration of action, making it a popular anesthetic agent among cataract surgeons.

Intraocular Anesthetic Agents

Intraocular anesthesia may be administered as an adjunct to topical anesthesia. Benzalkonium chloride is known to be toxic to the corneal endothelium, so agents injected intraocularly should be free of this preservative. Nonpreserved lidocaine 1% is generally the anesthetic agent injected intracamerally, but the use of preservative-free tetracaine has been reported.

REGIONAL ANESTHETIC AGENTS

Table 9.2 lists regional anesthetic agents in common use for ocular surgery. Combining local anesthetics is a common practice when providing regional ophthalmic anesthesia. Rapid-onset, short-acting agents like lidocaine or mepivacaine are frequently compounded with a long-acting, slow-onset agent like

Table 9.2. Regional Anesthetic Agents

Generic Name	Trade Name	Concentration (%)	Onset of Action (min)	Duration of Action (min)
Lidocaine	Xylocaine	1–4	4–6	40–60 120 (with epinephrine)
Mepivacaine	Carbocaine	1–2	3–5	120
Bupivacaine	Marcaine	0.25–0.75	5–11	480–720 (with epinephrine)
Etidocaine	Duranest	1–1.5	3	300–600

bupivacaine. The mixture combines the best properties of its constituents providing a fast onset of anesthesia and long duration of postoperative analgesia. When local anesthetics are mixed for injection, the final concentration of each constituent is diluted by the others. For example, a 1:1 mixture of lidocaine 4% and bupivacaine 0.75% produces a solution containing lidocaine 2% and bupivacaine 0.375%. The incidence of systemic toxicity with regional anesthesia relates to the drugs used, the total dosage administered, the vascularity of the injection site, and whether epinephrine was used as an adjuvant. Systemic toxicity with regional ophthalmic anesthesia is very rare, given the relatively small amount of anesthetic agent required for ophthalmic procedures.

Lidocaine

Lidocaine (Xylocaine) is commonly used in concentrations of 2% and 4% for regional anesthesia. It has a rapid onset of action and superb tissue penetration. The relatively short duration of action of lidocaine may be disadvantageous with prolonged ocular surgery, but its action may be extended by 75% or more with the addition of epinephrine.

Mepivacaine

Mepivacaine (Carbocaine) is generally used in a concentration of 2%. It has a clinical activity similar to lidocaine, but the duration of action of mepivacaine is about twice that of lidocaine because it has fewer vasodilatory properties.

Bupivacaine

Bupivacaine (Marcaine) in a concentration of 0.75% is typically used for regional ophthalmic anesthesia. It is a modified form of mepivacaine with a higher lipid solubility and protein-binding properties resulting in an increased potency and longer duration of action. The reduced tissue penetrance of bupivacaine delays its onset of action. Sodium bicarbonate will precipitate bupivacaine.

Etidocaine

Etidocaine (Duranest) is used in ophthalmic anesthesia typically in a 1.5% concentration. It is a modified form of lidocaine with a higher potency and a more prolonged duration of action. Unlike bupivacaine, etidocaine has a rapid onset of action. Because it couples fast onset and long duration of effect, etidocaine has become a popular local anesthetic agent in many ophthalmic practices.

Adjuvant Agents

Epinephrine, hyaluronidase, and sodium bicarbonate are adjuvant drugs that are commonly used to enhance the effect of regional anesthesia. Table 9.3 lists the constituents of a solution commonly used for regional anesthesia administered in a retrobulbar or peribulbar block.

Epinephrine

Epinephrine causes vasoconstriction at the site of injection, thereby delaying the absorption of regional anesthetic agents. The duration of action is prolonged for all except the longest-acting agents, and the effectiveness of the block is improved. The addition of 0.1 ml of 1:1000 epinephrine (100 µg) to 20 ml of regional anesthetic solution is standard, producing a concentration of 5 µg/ml (1:200,000).

Hyaluronidase

Hyaluronidase promotes the spread of the anesthetic solution through tissue. The enzyme causes a reversible hydrolysis of extracellular hyaluronic acid, breaking down collagen bonds and allowing the anesthetic to spread across fine connective tissue barriers. Hyaluronidase is typically added to the regional anesthetic injectant in a concentration of 7.5 units/ml.

Table 9.3. Anesthetic Solution Commonly Used For Regional Anesthesia

Amount	Generic Name
10 ml	Lidocaine 2–4%
10 ml	Bupivacaine 0.75%
0.1 ml	Epinephrine 1:200,000
150 units	Hyaluronidase
0.1 mEq	Sodium bicarbonate

Sodium Bicarbonate

Sodium bicarbonate augments the tissue penetrance and onset of action of local anesthetic agents by adjusting the pH of the solution toward the un-ionized basic form.

LOCAL ANESTHESIA

The use of topical and intraocular anesthesia involves appropriate patient selection and modification in surgical techniques.

Topical Anesthesia

With the advent of small-incision phacoemulsification cataract surgery, topical anesthesia has grown in popularity. Topical anesthesia provides anesthesia to the cornea, conjunctiva, and anterior sclera, but sensation is maintained in the eyelids, posterior sclera, intraocular tissues, and extraocular muscles. Therefore, when using topical anesthesia it is important to avoid excessive cautery, placement of a bridle suture, or manipulation of the iris. A modification in surgical technique is required when using topical anesthesia because sudden eye movements may be dangerous when instrumenting the eye. The surgeon should immobilize the globe using his or her nondominant hand whenever instruments are being used.

Appropriate patient selection is critical when considering topical anesthesia. A cooperative patient who is able to follow instructions during surgery is required. The patient's response to tonometry and A-scan ultrasonography appears to be a good predictor of how he or she will tolerate ocular surgery with this technique. Monocular patients may benefit from topical anesthesia because of their unique need for quick recovery of vision from the operated eye. Inappropriate candidates include patients who are very young, have a strong blink reflex, are unable to fixate (eg, because of macular degeneration), or have difficulty following commands (eg, because of dementia, deafness, or language barriers). Patients for whom surgery will be longer (more than 30 to 40 minutes) or difficult (eg, dense cataracts, small pupils, or weak zonules) are best managed with other forms of anesthesia.

Table 9.4 lists the advantages and disadvantages of topical anesthesia. The obvious advantage is avoidance of complications associated with injection into the orbit. Additionally, topical anesthesia eliminates the need to patch the eye after surgery because it avoids the temporary visual loss from the eye undergoing surgery. Furthermore, there is no need to interrupt anticoagulant or anti-

Table 9.4. Advantages and Disadvantages of Topical Anesthesia

Advantages	Avoids complications associated with orbital injection of anesthesia
	Eliminates the need to patch the eye after surgery
	Avoids the temporary loss of vision in the eye undergoing surgery
	No need to interrupt anticoagulant or antiplatelet therapy
Disadvantages	Patients are aware of surgical procedure
	Discomfort with the eyelid speculum and microscope light
	Pain associated with intraocular manipulation or IOP fluctuations
	Lack of akinesia
	Reliance on patient cooperation

platelet therapy. Disadvantages include patient awareness during the surgical procedure, discomfort with the eyelid speculum and microscope light, pain associated with intraocular manipulation or intraocular pressure fluctuation, lack of akinesia, and reliance on patient cooperation.

Delivery of Topical Anesthesia

An anesthetic agent is instilled topically onto the eye just before prepping the eye. The patient is instructed to fixate on the microscope light during the surgery to keep the eye stationary. Anesthetic drops are administered during the surgical procedure as needed. A variation of the technique involves placing pieces of Weck-cel or instrument wipe sponges (pledgets) saturated with anesthetic in the superior and inferior fornices. The pledgets are removed at the beginning or conclusion of the surgery. Sedative drugs can be helpful but are generally used minimally with topical anesthesia to allow retention of patient cooperation.

Intraocular Anesthesia

Intraocular anesthesia may be used in conjunction with topical anesthesia. The combination allows anesthesia of the cornea, conjunctiva, anterior sclera, iris, and ciliary body. The benefit of intraocular anesthesia is a reduction in pain associated with intraocular pressure fluctuation and manipulation of the iris, ciliary body, and lens. Patient selection is the same as for surgery performed under topical anesthesia alone.

Delivery of Intraocular Anesthesia

Nonpreserved lidocaine 1% is irrigated into the anterior chamber through a paracentesis or side-port incision. Directing the drug posterior to the iris during injection may provide a maximal effect on the iris and ciliary body. After 15 to 30 seconds, the anesthetic is washed out by irrigation of balanced salt solution or viscoelastic (see the review of intraocular fluids in Chapter 10). A transient decrease in vision may occur if the anesthetic reaches the retina.

REGIONAL ANESTHESIA

Regional anesthesia for intraocular surgery involves the injection of anesthetic agents into the orbit to provide anesthesia to the cornea, conjunctiva, sclera, intraocular structures, and extraocular muscles. Retrobulbar, peribulbar, and parabulbar blocks are the common methods to deliver regional anesthesia. There is little or no patient sensitivity to intraocular pressure fluctuations and to the microscope light with regional anesthesia. Extraocular motility is eliminated, so there is less need for patient cooperation to control eye movements. Regional anesthesia is especially suited for patients who are anxious and for those with mental or psychological disorders. Surgical procedures that require extensive intraocular manipulation or are expected to be lengthy (more than 30 to 40 minutes in duration) are best performed with regional anesthesia.

Table 9.5 lists the advantages and disadvantages of regional anesthesia. Regional anesthesia offers the advantages of full anesthesia and akinesia of the eye, reduced reliance on patient cooperation, and suitability for surgical procedures of relatively greater complexity and longer duration. Disadvantages of this technique for ocular anesthesia include the need to patch the eye during the postoperative period of recovery from anesthesia, advisability of interrupting anticoagulant or antiplatelet therapy, and potential complications associated with the orbital injection of anesthesia.

Table 9.5. Advantages and Disadvantages of Regional Anesthesia

Advantages	Full anesthesia and akinesia of the eye
	Reduced reliance on patient cooperation
	Suitable for surgical procedures of relatively greater complexity and longer duration
Disadvantages	Need to patch the eye during postoperative period of recovery from anesthesia
	Advisable to interrupt anticoagulant and antiplatelet therapy
	Complications associated with orbital injection of anesthesia

Retrobulbar Block

In a retrobulbar block, anesthetic solution is injected into the space behind the globe within the muscle cone of the four rectus muscles. A 1.25-inch, 25- or 27-gauge needle is inserted transcutaneously or transconjunctivally just above the inferior orbital rim at a point in line with the lateral limbus (Figure 9.1). A short-beveled, blunt needle (Atkinson's) can be used to reduce the risk of scleral perforation and retrobulbar hemorrhage. A sharp disposable needle produces less injection pain and is safe when proper injection technique is employed. The patient should be in primary gaze; an upward and inward gaze should be avoided because it places the optic nerve in a more vulnerable position. During needle entry, an index fingertip may be positioned between the globe and orbital rim to elevate the eye. The needle is advanced tangential to the globe and parallel to the bony floor of the orbit.

Once the equator of the globe is passed, the needle is redirected upward and medially into the muscle cone. Increased resistance or globe rotation during needle advancement could indicate engagement of the sclera; if either is detected, the needle should be repositioned. It has been suggested that the needle should not be inserted more than 31 mm from the orbital rim, and the midsagittal plane of the eye should not be crossed because the optic nerve lies on the nasal side of this plane. After aspiration to ensure that the needle tip is not in a blood vessel, 3 to 4 ml of anesthetic solution is injected slowly. As the needle is withdrawn, orbicularis oculi muscle akinesia may be achieved by injecting 1 to 2 ml of anesthetic anterior to the orbital septum.

After injection, orbital compression is maintained for several minutes using manual compression or a mechanical compression device (eg, Honan's balloon) to assist in the spread of anesthesia. While orbital compression has been used safely for many years, it has been implicated as a cause of ptosis and impaired retinal circulation in case reports.

After about 5 minutes, an assessment of globe movement and orbicularis function is made. If akinesia is inadequate, a supplemental injection may be given. Small rotational movements of the globe are commonly seen. The motor nerves to the four rectus muscles and inferior oblique access their respective muscle bellies within the muscle cone, whereas the trochlear nerve remains outside the cone and enters the superior oblique at its superolateral edge. This anatomic difference explains the limited akinesia of the superior oblique after a retrobulbar block.

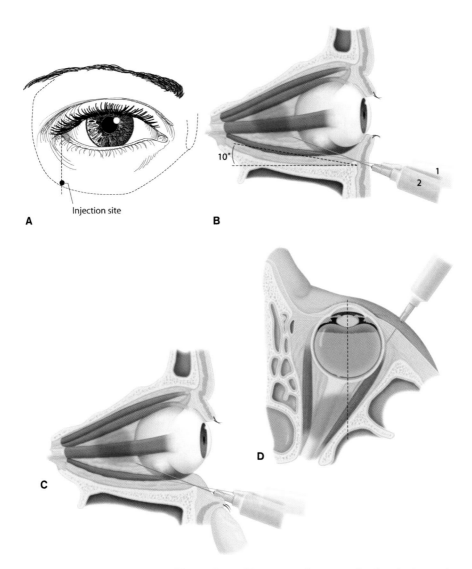

Figure 9.1. Retrobulbar block. A 1.25-inch, 25- or 27-gauge needle is inserted at the inferotemporal orbital rim at a point in line with the lateral limbus (A). The needle is advanced tangential to the globe and parallel to the bony floor of the orbit, which inclines at an angle of 10° from the transverse plane (B1). Once the equator of the globe is passed, the needle is redirected upward and medially into the muscle cone (B2). Either a transcutaneous (B) or transconjunctival (C) approach may be used. The midsagittal plane of the eye should not be crossed because the optic nerve lies on the nasal side of this plane (D). (Illustration by Mark M. Miller)

Peribulbar Block

A peribulbar block involves injection of anesthetic solution within the orbit, but outside the muscle cone. A 1-inch, 25- or 27-gauge, blunt-tipped

(Atkinson's) or sharp disposable needle is inserted in the same transcutaneous or transconjunctival location as described for a retrobulbar block (Figure 9.2). The needle is advanced tangential to the eye with penetration 3 to 4 mm posterior to the equator of the globe. After aspiration, 4 to 8 ml of anesthetic solution is injected slowly. Akinesia of the orbicularis muscle can be achieved by injecting 1 to 2 ml of anesthetic into the lower lid anterior to the orbital septum. Pressure is applied to the eye using manual compression or a mechanical compression device (eg, Honan's balloon). Globe motility and eyelid function are evaluated after 10 to 20 minutes.

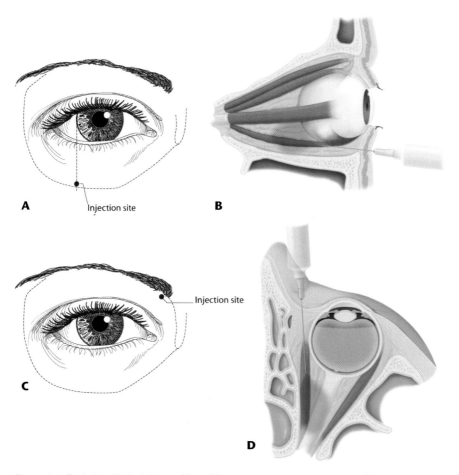

Figure 9.2. Peribulbar block. A 1-inch, 25- or 27-gauge needle is inserted at the inferotemporal orbital rim at a point in line with the lateral limbus (A). The needle is advanced tangential to the globe and parallel to the orbital floor with penetration 3 to 4 mm posterior to the equator (B). If necessary, an additional injection may be made in the upper eyelid at a point midway between the medial canthus and supraorbital notch (C). The needle is advanced tangential to the globe to the equator (D). (Illustration by Mark M. Miller)

If necessary, an additional injection may be made in the upper eyelid at a point midway between the medial canthus and supraorbital notch at a point in line with the medial limbus. The needle is advanced tangential to the globe to the equator, and an additional 2 to 3 ml of anesthetic solution is injected after aspiration. Only 15% to 20% of peribulbar blocks require an upper lid injection to supplement a lower lid injection. There is a greater risk of ptosis and scleral perforation with upper lid injections.

Many surgeons have abandoned the retrobulbar block in favor of the peribulbar block. The major advantage of the peribulbar block over the retrobulbar block is the reduced risk of complications such as retrobulbar hemorrhage, scleral perforation, central nervous system anesthesia, and optic nerve damage. In patients with high myopia and a long axial length (which may increase the risk of globe perforation with more posterior injection), it is prudent to use a peribulbar block or general anesthesia rather than a retrobulbar block. The disadvantage of the peribulbar technique is a slower onset of anesthesia, the need for a larger total volume of injected anesthetic solution, and the frequent requirement for supplemental injections.

Parabulbar Block

A parabulbar block entails injection of anesthetic solution into the anterior intraconal space using a blunt cannula after dissection into the sub-Tenon's space. After administration of topical anesthesia, an incision is made through conjunctiva and Tenon's capsule. A blunt metal or flexible cannula is introduced into the sub-Tenon's space, and the tip is passed posteriorly beyond the equator of the globe (Figure 9.3). Local anesthetic solution is injected; the degree of akinesia and anesthesia is proportional to the volume of anesthetic used. Disadvantages of this technique include an increased incidence of conjunctival chemosis and hemorrhage, risk of damage to the vortex veins, and a frequent need for supplementation.

GENERAL ANESTHESIA

In the elderly population, the advantages of regional anesthesia usually outweigh those of general anesthesia for the performance of safe and comfortable surgery in a cost-effective manner. While the incidences of death and major complications are similar between general and regional anesthesia, general anesthesia has been reported to produce more postoperative nausea and vomiting, intraoperative oxygen desaturation and hemodynamic fluctuation, and

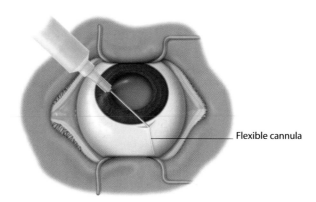

Figure 9.3. Parabulbar block. A blunt metal or flexible cannula is introduced into the sub-Tenon's space and passed posteriorly beyond the equator of the globe. (Illustration by Mark M. Miller)

Flexible cannula

initial postoperative pain. Therefore, it is prudent to avoid general anesthesia in patients with severe cardiovascular or pulmonary disease if possible.

General anesthesia in ophthalmology is typically used in pediatric strabismus surgery and lengthy vitreoretinal procedures. Additionally, patients who cannot cooperate adequately (eg, children or people with tremor, inability to lie supine or severe mental or psychological impairment) may not be candidates for regional anesthesia in any surgical procedure. Patients who have experienced a prior complication with regional anesthesia (eg, retrobulbar hemorrhage, inadvertent intrathecal injection of anesthetic) should have subsequent ocular surgery under general anesthesia. Lengthy ocular procedures (more than 3 to 4 hours) are best performed with general anesthesia.

Table 9.6 lists the advantages and disadvantages of general anesthesia. General anesthesia offers the advantages of complete control of the patient, avoidance of complications associated with orbital injection, and application to patients in all age groups. Disadvantages of general anesthesia include absence of postoperative analgesia, an increased incidence of postoperative nausea and vomiting, greater intraoperative cardiovascular and pulmonary stress, a risk of malignant hyperthermia, slower immediate postoperative recovery, and greater cost.

The main requirements for general anesthesia in ocular surgery are anesthesia and akinesia of the globe and eyelids and control of the intraocular pressure (to protect against extrusion of intraocular contents). A variety of inhalation and intravenous agents may be used to accomplish these goals. Following a smooth induction, a deep level of anesthesia is maintained until the wound has been closed. A depolarizing muscle relaxant is commonly administered while the eye is open. Intraoperative use of antiemetics decreases the incidence of postoperative nausea and vomiting.

Table 9.6. Advantages and Disadvantages of General Anesthesia

Advantages	Complete control of patient
	Avoids complications associated with orbital injection
	Applicable to all ages
Disadvantages	Absence of postoperative analgesia
	More postoperative nausea and vomiting
	Greater cardiovascular and pulmonary stress
	Risk of malignant hyperthermia
	Slower immediate postoperative recovery
	More expensive

Ocular complications associated with general anesthesia for eye surgery are usually related to coughing and straining during surgery or nausea and vomiting in the postoperative period. Sudden changes in intraocular pressure may lead to suprachoroidal hemorrhage, wound dehiscence, or vitreous loss. Most intravenous and inhalation anesthetics used in general anesthesia produce a reduction in intraocular pressure. The use of nitrous oxide gas should be discontinued at least 20 minutes before intravitreal gas injection (SF_6, C_3F_8) during vitreoretinal procedures. Nitrous oxide rapidly enters the gas bubble, producing an increase in its size and intraocular pressure elevation.

FACIAL NERVE BLOCKS

Contraction of the orbicularis oculi muscle (innervated by branches of the facial nerve) causes eyelid closure. Following orbital injection of an anesthetic agent and hyaluronidase, spread of the agent anteriorly through the orbital septum typically produces akinesia of the orbicularis oculi muscle. Therefore, facial nerve blocks are generally not required when a retrobulbar or peribulbar block is administered. In the rare cases when eyelid squeezing is still present, a facial nerve block may prove useful. Various techniques for facial nerve blocks (including the Van Lint block, O'Brien block, and Nadbath-Ellis block) have been developed.

Van Lint Block

The Van Lint block involves infiltrating anesthesia in the region of the terminal branches of the facial nerve. A 1.5-inch, 25-gauge disposable needle is inserted

1 cm lateral to the lateral orbital rim (Figure 9.4A). After aspiration, 1 to 2 ml of anesthetic solution is injected deeply on the periosteum. The needle is withdrawn slightly and redirected along the inferior orbital margin injecting 1 to 2 ml of anesthetic outside the orbital rim. The needle is withdrawn to the original entry site and redirected along the superior orbital margin injecting an additional 1 to 2 ml of anesthetic solution.

O'Brien Block

The O'Brien block produces akinesia of the orbicularis oculi muscle by anesthetizing the facial nerve at its proximal trunk. The condyloid process of the mandible is palpated in front of the tragus. By asking the patient to open and close his or her mouth, the condyloid process may be felt moving forward under the finger. A 1-inch, 27-gauge disposable needle is inserted at the center of the condyloid process to the periosteum (Figure 9.4B). After aspiration, 3 ml of anesthetic solution is injected.

Figure 9.4. Facial nerve blocks. (A) Van Lint block. (B). O'Brien block. (C) Nadbath-Ellis block. (Illustration by Mark M. Miller)

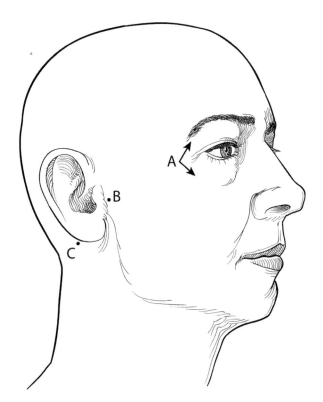

Nadbath-Ellis Block

The Nadbath-Ellis block involves injection of anesthetic solution in the region where the facial nerve emerges from the stylomastoid foramen. The tympano-mastoid fissure is palpated at the anterosuperior border of the mastoid process, where it fuses with the tympanic portion of the temporal bone. The area may be felt as a convexity below the external auditory meatus and behind the pinna. A 5/8-inch, 25- or 26-gauge disposable needle is inserted into the tympano-mastoid fissure (Figure 9.4C). After aspiration, 1 to 2 ml of anesthetic solution is injected. The injection should be made with the head turned to the opposite side to pull the sternocleidomastoid muscle out of the area, and with the mouth closed to widen the space between the mandible and mastoid process.

COMPLICATIONS OF OPHTHALMIC ANESTHESIA

Possible complications of ophthalmic anesthesia include those associated with orbital injection, the oculocardiac reflex, and malignant hyperthermia.

Complications of Orbital Injection

Complications as a result of injection of anesthesia into the orbit include retrobulbar hemorrhage, scleral perforation, spread of anesthetic into the central nervous system, and strabismus.

Retrobulbar Hemorrhage
Retrobulbar hemorrhages vary in severity, but they generally present with sub-conjunctival hemorrhage, eyelid ecchymosis, proptosis, and elevated intraocular pressure. Venous hemorrhages usually spread slowly and are limited, while arterial hemorrhages develop rapidly and can be massive. Vascular compromise to the optic nerve and retina may result. The incidence of serious retrobulbar bleeding has been reported as 1% to 3%. The intraocular pressure should be monitored after a retrobulbar hemorrhage, and treatment should be instituted with aqueous suppressants, a hyperosmotic agent, and lateral canthotomy and cantholysis as needed. The surgical procedure should be cancelled when a serious retrobulbar hemorrhage has occurred.

Scleral Perforation
It is imperative that proper technique be used when administering regional anesthetic blocks to minimize the risk of scleral perforation. There is a greater

risk of globe perforation in myopic eyes, a superior injection, improper needle insertion, and use of long (1.5-inch), sharp needles. Scleral perforation is a complication occurring in 1 in 1,300 to 12,000 retrobulbar and peribulbar blocks. It may manifest with immediate ocular pain with injection, hypotony, poor red reflex, and vitreous hemorrhage. The planned surgery should be cancelled if this complication occurs, and immediate consultation with a vitreo-retinal specialist arranged, to evaluate the retina for tears and detachment.

Central Nervous System Spread of Anesthesia

A potentially lethal complication of regional anesthetic blocks is the central nervous system (CNS) spread of anesthetic along the optic nerve dural sheath into the subarachnoid space, pons, and midbrain. The incidence of this complication is 1 in 350 to 500 patients. CNS spread of anesthesia should be suspected with symptoms of mental confusion, shivering, seizures, nausea or vomiting, dysphagia, sudden swings in cardiovascular vital signs, or respiratory depression. There may be amaurosis, extraocular muscle paresis, and pupillary dilation in the contralateral eye.

Symptoms of brainstem anesthesia usually develop within 2 to 30 minutes of retrobulbar injection, and they may last for 30 minutes or several hours. This complication emphasizes the need for a standby anesthesiologist when administering regional ocular anesthesia and a favorable outcome is usually observed when immediate support is provided. To prevent the CNS spread of anesthesia, deep orbital injection should be avoided and the eye should be maintained in primary gaze during the block. When the eye is turned upward and inward, the optic nerve and nerve sheath are in a more vulnerable position to the retrobulbar needle.

Strabismus

Strabismus may develop after injection of regional anesthesia into the orbit. Persistent extraocular muscle dysfunction and diplopia is common during the first 24 to 48 hours postoperatively, especially when large volumes of long-acting anesthetic agents are used. Permanent strabismus may occur if fusion cannot be recovered after disruption by the anesthesia, due to pre-existing conditions such as thyroid eye disease, myasthenia gravis, cranial nerve palsies, or prolonged visual deprivation from a cataract. Animal and human studies have demonstrated myotoxicity of local anesthetic agents, particularly when injected into muscle bellies. The inferior rectus muscle is most often affected. Persistent diplopia may be treated with prism or strabismus surgery.

Oculocardiac Reflex

The oculocardiac reflex (OCR) is stimulated when traction on extraocular muscles produces vagal effects on the heart via a trigeminal-vagal reflex. Direct pressure on the globe, orbital anesthetic injection, and elevation of intraocular pressure may also elicit this reflex. Cardiac manifestations of the OCR include bradycardia, ectopic beats, nodal rhythms, atrioventricular block, and even cardiac arrest. The OCR is most commonly observed with strabismus surgery, but it may occur with other ocular procedures (eg, enucleation, retinal surgery) under either local or general anesthesia. Therefore, EKG monitoring should be performed continuously during all ophthalmic surgeries. The surgeon should immediately stop manipulating the eye or its muscles when an arrhythmia occurs. The OCR fatigues easily, and usually there is little or no activity after a brief pause in surgical stimuli. When OCR is severe, it may be treated with intravenous atropine.

Malignant Hyperthermia

Malignant hyperthermia is a rare disorder of skeletal muscle metabolism that can be triggered by succinylcholine and the inhalation anesthetics halothane, enflurane, and isoflurane. Its incidence has been estimated as 1 in 15,000, and patients with muscle abnormalities like strabismus and ptosis are thought to be at greater risk for developing it. The disorder is inherited in an autosomal dominant pattern. Before strabismus surgery, it is important to inquire about previous anesthetic problems in both parents and their families.

Malignant hyperthermia presents with tachycardia, tachypnea, hypercarbia, muscle spasm, severe acidosis, and a rapid rise in body temperature; the ophthalmic surgeon should be aware of these early manifestations, as early recognition may be life-saving. Upon recognition of malignant hyperthermia, anesthetic agents should be discontinued, hyperventilation with oxygen started, and treatment with dantrolene begun. Surgery should be terminated as soon as possible, even if the procedure is not complete.

KEY POINTS

→ The most commonly used topical ophthalmic anesthetic agents are proparacaine 0.5% and tetracaine 0.5%.

→ The most commonly used regional ophthalmic anesthetic agents are lidocaine (Xylocaine) 2% to 4%, mepivacaine (Carbocaine) 2%, bupivacaine (Marcaine) 0.75%, and etidocaine (Duranest) 1.5%.

→ Epinephrine (1:1000) and hyaluronidase are often added to regional anesthesia solutions to enhance activity.

→ Common regional ophthalmic anesthetic techniques include retrobulbar or peribulbar injection and facial nerve blocks.

→ Potential complications from orbital injection include orbital hemorrhage, scleral perforation, CNS spread of anesthesia, and strabismus.

→ General anesthesia in ophthalmology is typically used in pediatric strabismus surgery and lengthy vitreoretinal procedures, and in patients who cannot cooperate adequately for local anesthesia.

SELF-ASSESSMENT TEST

1. A rapid-onset, short-acting anesthetic agent like lidocaine is frequently combined with a long-acting, slow-onset agent like bupivacaine for regional anesthesia by orbital injection. (true or false)

2. Which of the following agents is routinely added to anesthetic solution to enhance regional anesthesia?
   a. Hyaluronidase
   b. Sodium chloride
   c. Atropine
   d. Cocaine

3. When administering a retrobulbar block, the patient should be instructed to look upward and inward. (true or false)

4. Which of the following would make a patient a poor candidate for topical anesthesia? (list all that apply)
   a. Demented
   b. Deaf
   c. Strong blink reflex
   d. All of the above

5. Which of the following patients should have their ocular procedure performed under general anesthesia? (list all that apply)
   a. 6-month-old infant undergoing strabismus surgery
   b. 50-year-old man undergoing a lengthy vitreoretinal procedure
   c. 72-year-old woman undergoing cataract surgery after her prior surgery was cancelled due to a retrobulbar hemorrhage during the retrobulbar block
   d. All of the above

6. During general anesthesia, nitrous oxide should be discontinued at least 20 minutes before injection of C_3F_8 or SF_6 gas into the vitreous cavity. (true or false)

7. It is best to avoid a retrobulbar block in highly myopic eyes with a long axial length. (true or false)

For preferred responses to these questions, see pages 223–224.

SUGGESTED READING

Ahn JC, Stanley JA. Subarachnoid injection as a complication of retrobulbar anesthesia. *Am J Ophthalmol.* 1987;103:225–230.

Britton B, Hervey R, Kasten K, et al. Intraocular irritation evaluation of benzalkonium chloride in rabbits. *Ophthalmic Surg.* 1976;7:46–55.

Donlon JV. Anesthesia for ophthalmic surgery. In: Albert DM, Jakobiec FA, et al, eds. *Principles and Practice of Ophthalmology.* Philadelphia: WB Saunders Co, 1994; v 5, chap 231.

Duker JS, Belmont JB, Benson WE, et al. Inadvertent globe perforations during retrobulbar and peribulbar anesthesia. Patient characteristics, surgical management, and visual outcome. *Ophthalmology.* 1991;98:519–526.

Fanning GL. Monitored sedation for ophthalmic surgery. In: Kumar CM, Doods C, Fanning GL, eds. *Ophthalmic Anesthesia.* Lisse, The Netherlands: Swets & Zeitlinger, 2002; chap 7.

Fraser SG, Siriwadena D, Jamieson H, et al. Indicators of patient suitability for topical anesthesia. *J Cataract Refract Surg.* 1997;23:781–783.

Hamilton RC, Gimbel HV, Strunin L. Regional anaesthesia for 12,000 cataract extraction and intraocular lens implantation procedures. *Can J Anaesth*. 1988;35:615–623.

Katsev DA, Drews RC, Rose BT. An anatomic study of retrobulbar needle path length. *Ophthalmology*. 1989;96:1221–1224.

Lynch S, Wolf GL, Berlin I. General anesthesia for cataract surgery: a comparative review of 2217 consecutive cases. *Anesth Analg*. 1974;53:909–913.

Morgan CM, Schatz H, Vine AK, et al. Ocular complications associated with retrobulbar injections. *Ophthalmology*. 1988;95:660–665.

Nicoll JM, Acharya PA, Ahlen K, et al. Central nervous system complications after 6000 retrobulbar blocks. *Anesth Analg*. 1987;66:1298–1302.

Rainin EA, Carlson BM. Postoperative diplopia and ptosis. A clinical hypothesis based on the myotoxicity of local anesthetics. *Arch Ophthalmol*. 1985;103:1337–1339.

Rosenthal KJ. Deep, topical, nerve-block anesthesia. *J Cataract Refract Surg*. 1995;21:499–503.

Stead SW, Miller KM. Anesthesia for ophthalmic surgery. In: Spaeth GL, ed. *Ophthalmic Surgery: Principles and Practice*. Philadelphia: WB Saunders & Co, 2003; chap 2.

Unsold R, Stanley JA, DeGroot J. The CT-topography of retrobulbar anesthesia. Anatomic-clinical correlation of complications and suggestion of a modified technique. *Albrecht von Graefes Arch Klin Exp Ophthalmol*. 1981;217:125–136.

Chapter 10

Intraocular Fluids

James P. Dunn, MD

The use of intraocular fluids in anterior segment surgery is essential in providing effective working space, control of tissue, appropriate pupil size, and control of surgical instruments for the surgeon. This chapter helps the beginning resident understand when, how, and why to use these fluids in order to make cataract and glaucoma surgery safer and more effective.

Intraocular fluids can be classified into six categories: viscoelastics; irrigating fluids; mydriatics and miotics; anesthetics; corticosteroids, antibiotics, and antifungals; and capsular staining agents.

VISCOELASTICS

Viscoelastics are gel-like materials that protect delicate intraocular structures, maintain space, and allow manipulation of crystalline and intraocular lenses. All viscoelastics share the desirable property of pseudoplasticity; that is, they assume a gel-like configuration at low shear rates (such as occurs during capsulorrhexis or lens cracking) but change to a more liquid solution at high shear rates (as occurs during phacoemulsification and aspiration). These materials are commonly classified as either *cohesive* or *dispersive*. Most viscoelastics are composed of hyaluronic acid of varying molecular weight (cohesive) or a combination of hyaluronic acid and chondroitin sulfate (dispersive). Hydroxypropyl methylcellulose 2% is another dispersive viscoelastic.

In general, cohesive viscoelastics are better at maintaining space and are more easily removed at the end of surgery. However, they are also more easily removed during phacoemulsification itself, thereby possibly jeopardizing endothelial cell protection in prolonged surgery or in eyes with small anterior chambers (as in hyperopia). In addition, cohesive viscoelastics tend to "drag" adjacent tissue with them during removal, including iris or vitreous. Dispersive viscoelastics are better at coating tissue and may provide more prolonged endothelial cell protection. However, they are less easily removed than cohesive viscoelastics, because they tend to "fragment" upon removal. Consequently, they may be more likely to induce elevated intraocular pressure in the first 24 hours after cataract surgery. They are also more likely to produce bubbles when injected into the eye, which can compromise the surgeon's view.

There is no "perfect" viscoelastic, and the beginning surgeon should try to gain experience with both cohesive and dispersive types. Indeed, some surgeons prefer to use both types for "high-risk" eyes, such as those with borderline endothelial functioning, dense nuclei requiring high amounts of phaco energy for removal, or weak zonules. The so-called "soft shell" technique involves first injecting a dispersive viscoelastic into the anterior chamber (Figure 10.1), followed by a more posterior injection of a cohesive viscoelastic. The cohesive viscoelastic pushes the dispersive viscoelastic up against the corneal endothelium, where it theoretically remains during surgery.

Figure 10.1. Ring of dispersive viscoelastic pushed up against endothelium by injection of cohesive viscoelastic. (Illustration by Mark M. Miller)

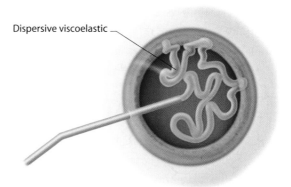

Dispersive viscoelastic

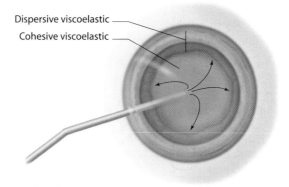

Dispersive viscoelastic
Cohesive viscoelastic

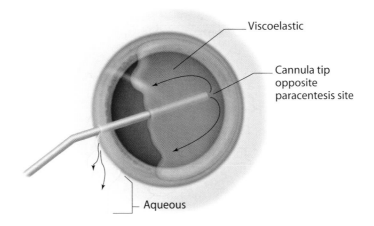

Figure 10.2. Injection of viscoelastic into the eye through a small-bore cannula. Note placement of the cannula tip opposite the site of entry, injecting the viscoelastic so that it fills the anterior chamber and forces aqueous out of the eye. (Illustration by Mark M. Miller)

Viscoelastics are injected into the eye through a small-bore cannula, usually just prior to the creation of the corneal or scleral wound. The tip of the cannula should be placed opposite the site of entry, injecting the viscoelastic so that it fills the anterior chamber and forces aqueous out of the eye (Figure 10.2). Underfilling the anterior chamber prior to the phacoemulsification incision results in a soft eye that tends to collapse and can result in a wound length longer than is desired. Overfilling the anterior chamber steepens the corneal curvature and can result in an incision length shorter than is desired. Hydroxypropyl methylcellulose can also be used to coat the corneal surface, obviating the need for frequent irrigation by the assistant during surgery.

Cohesive Viscoelastics

Cohesive viscoelastics are most useful in maintaining anterior chamber space. They can help maximally flatten the anterior lens capsule, which reduces the tendency for the capsular tear to "run downhill" and extend peripherally during capsulorrhexis, and should be used liberally in this stage of cataract surgery. They can also push away and flatten the capsule, which can sometimes fold up accordion-like and impair the surgeon's view of the leading edge of the capsulorrhexis (Figure 10.3). When a bent needle is used to perform capsulorrhexis (as opposed to a Utrata forceps), it is highly recommended that the needle be attached to a cohesive viscoelastic syringe. Cohesive viscoelastics

Figure 10.3. Use of viscoelastic pushed up against endothelium by injection of cohesive viscoelastic. (Illustration by Mark M. Miller)

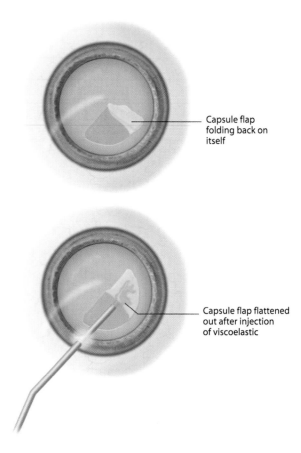

Capsule flap folding back on itself

Capsule flap flattened out after injection of viscoelastic

are also helpful in dilating a small pupil (often in combination with various mechanical pupil-stretching techniques), in maintaining maximal separation of nuclear sections to facilitate lens cracking, in manipulating lens fragments out of the capsular bag for phacoemulsification in the iris plane, and in expanding the capsular bag prior to intraocular lens placement. Another useful role of cohesive viscoelastics is in "viscodissection." In this technique, subincisional cortex which is difficult to remove can be separated from the posterior capsule and pushed into the peripheral capsular bag (Figure 10.4), where it can be more safely and easily aspirated after placement of the intraocular lens.

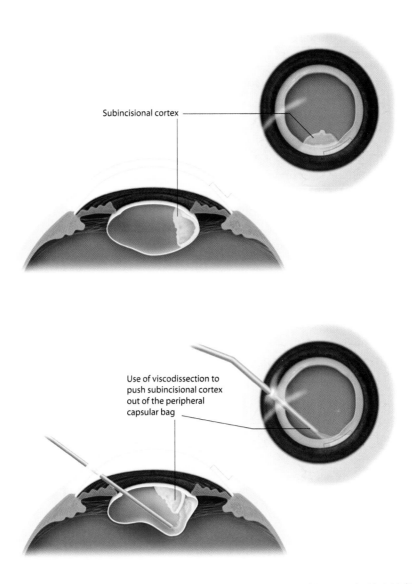

Figure 10.4. Technique of viscodissection to loosen subincisional cortex. (Illustration by Mark M. Miller)

Dispersive Viscoelastics

On the other hand, the tendency of a dispersive viscoelastic to fragment upon removal can be used to the surgeon's advantage if there is a capsular tear or zonular dehiscence; tamponading the area with a dispersive viscoelastic may allow the surgeon to remove adjacent cortex without dragging vitreous into the aspiration tip.

Dispersive viscoelastics may provide more prolonged corneal endothelial cell protection than cohesive viscoelastics, and they are often recommended for cases in which the lens nucleus is especially dense (requiring higher phaco energy for removal), the anterior chamber is shallow (reducing the space between the phaco tip and the corneal endothelium), or there is preexisting compromise of the corneal endothelium.

Removing Viscoelastics

Viscoelastics should be removed completely at the end of cataract surgery, because retained viscoelastic will clog the trabecular meshwork and can cause marked elevation in intraocular pressure for 24 to 48 hours after surgery. Such pressure spikes can cause pain and corneal edema. Some surgeons prefer to leave a small amount of viscoelastic in the eye at the end of trabeculectomy surgery to reduce the risk of chamber shallowing in the first 24 to 48 hours postoperatively. Cohesive viscoelastics can be removed more quickly than dispersive viscoelastics, since the former tend to coalesce into a large bolus during aspiration. To remove the material completely, the surgeon may need to place the irrigation/aspiration tip behind the lens implant, or to rock the lens from side to side while aspirating. Retained viscoelastic may also cause capsular distension syndrome, in which the viscoelastic causes osmotic flow of aqueous into the capsular bag behind the intraocular lens, which pushes the lens forward and causes a myopic shift.

IRRIGATING FLUIDS

Irrigating fluid is necessary in phacoemulsification to cool the phaco tip and prevent wound burn. The basic intraoperative irrigating fluid is balanced salt solution. The addition of 0.5 ml of epinephrine 1:1000 diluted 1:10 may help enhance pupillary dilation and reduce bleeding when lysis of posterior synechiae is required. The addition of glutathione (BSS Plus) may provide better endothelial cell protection than balanced salt solution alone. Finally, antibiotics such as vancomycin 20 mcg/ml are sometimes added to reduce the risk of endophthalmitis. Keep in mind that controlled clinical trials have not demonstrated a reduction in postoperative endophthalmitis with the use intraocular antibiotics, and any potential benefit must be weighed against possible toxicity, including cystoid macular edema and endothelial damage (especially if a dilutional error is made in adding the antibiotic). Some clinicians recommend using chilled irrigating solution in eyes with compromised endothelial function. In all circumstances, the surgeon should strive to minimize the volume of irrigating solution used during surgery, since the turbulence of flow within the eye may damage endothelial cells. The irrigating ports of the phaco and irrigation/aspiration handpieces should be directed away from the endothelium during surgery.

MYDRIATICS AND MIOTICS

The use of epinephrine in the irrigating fluid to enhance dilation and reduce bleeding is discussed in the previous section. Before injection of viscoelastic, 0.5 ml of preservative-free epinephrine 1:1000 diluted 1:10 with balanced salt solution may also be injected directly into the anterior chamber for the same purposes.

Intracameral miotics are used in glaucoma surgery to constrict the pupil to facilitate creation of an iridectomy, in corneal transplant surgery to help protect the crystalline lens during trephination, and in cataract surgery to prevent iris capture of the intraocular lens. Miotics are also helpful in identifying vitreous strands that may be extending to the wound margin after capsular ruptures (Figure 10.5), and they may help reduce the risk of postoperative pressure spikes. Miotics are usually unnecessary in routine cataract surgery if the intraocular lens is completely covered by the anterior capsular rim. Furthermore, miotics are potentially pro-inflammatory, and for this reason are best avoided if possible following surgery for uveitic cataracts.

The two miotics commercially available are acetylcholine 1% (Miochol) and carbachol 0.01% (Miostat). Both are direct-acting parasympathomimetics. About 0.5 ml is an adequate volume for injection. Acetylcholine causes pupillary constriction within seconds but lasts only several hours, while carbachol may take 2 to 5 minutes to induce miosis but may last up to 24 hours. Both miotics will also reduce intraocular pressure. Carbachol will therefore provide more sustained intraocular pressure control, but it will also result in a small pupil on the first postoperative day, making visualization of the retina more difficult.

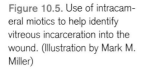

Figure 10.5. Use of intracameral miotics to help identify vitreous incarceration into the wound. (Illustration by Mark M. Miller)

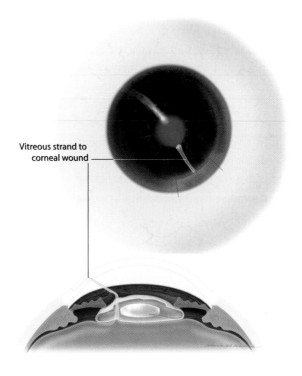

Vitreous strand to corneal wound

ANESTHETICS

Intracameral anesthetics are sometimes used to supplement topical anesthetics in cataract surgery. Their use may reduce the discomfort patients can feel when there is stretching of the ciliary body, as occurs when going to foot position 1 in phacoemulsification. Preservative-free lidocaine 1% must be used, because the preservatives may cause severe corneal endothelial damage (the use of preservative-free tetracaine has been reported). The injection (no more than 0.5 ml) is usually given prior to injection of the viscoelastic.

CORTICOSTEROIDS, ANTIBIOTICS, AND ANTIFUNGALS

Intracameral antibiotics and antifungals are usually given only as intravitreous injections following open globe repair or as treatment for presumed endophthalmitis. The drug is injected through a pars plana incision 3 to 4 mm posterior to the limbus, using a 30-gauge needle. Typical regimens include amphotericin 5 to 10 mcg in 0.05 to 0.1 ml, vancomycin 1.0 mg in 0.1 ml, clindamycin

1.0 mg in 0.1 ml, and ceftazidime 2.25 mg in 0.1 ml. While some clinicians favor the use of antibiotic injections in the anterior chamber following cataract surgery to help prevent endophthalmitis, most surgeons feel that the potential risk of endothelial damage outweighs any potential benefit, and their use in this manner is generally discouraged. Aminoglycosides in particular are toxic to the retina and should not be used.

Intravitreous injections of corticosteroids in the form of dexamethasone sodium phosphate or triamcinolone acetonide have been used recently to help treat or prevent cystoid macular edema due to uveitis or following surgery, and to treat choroidal neovascularization. While limited publications have shown considerable benefit, controlled studies are lacking, and caution is recommended. Triamcinolone acetonide preparations contain various preservatives and inactive ingredients that can cause a sterile endophthalmitis. True infectious endophthalmitis has also been reported, and sterilization of the conjunctiva with povidone-iodine solution prior to intraocular injection is mandatory. Intravitreous dexamethasone 400 mcg in 0.1 ml may also be useful in reducing inflammation in cases of gram-positive endophthalmitis.

CAPSULAR STAINING AGENTS

In cases of dense white cataracts, staining the anterior capsule greatly enhances visualization of the capsulorrhexis. Indocyanine green 0.5% is commonly used by surgeons for this purpose, although such usage is not FDA-approved. The diluted solution is injected underneath an air bubble and allowed to stay in place for 20 to 30 seconds, and then is exchanged for balanced salt solution or viscoelastic. It often helps to inject a small amount of viscoelastic just inside the paracentesis before injecting the air bubble; the viscoelastic helps keep the air bubble inside the eye as the dye is injected. Small pupils must be dilated prior to injection of the dye, as only the exposed anterior lens capsule will take up the stain.

Trypan blue 0.06% is another dye used to stain the capsule, and may be more effective than indocyanine green. It is available in the United States as VisionBlue trypan blue ophthalmic solution (Dutch Ophthalmic USA, Kingston, New Hampshire).

KEY POINTS

→ Viscoelastics are primarily composed of hyaluronic acid.

→ Cohesive viscoelastics fragment less, are better for maintaining space in the eye, and are more easily removed.

→ Dispersive viscoelastics fragment more and provide better coating of the corneal endothelium, but are more difficult to remove from the eye.

→ Intracameral miotics acetylcholine and carbachol may be used to identify vitreous strands, protect the lens in penetrating keratoplasty, facilitate iridectomy, and prevent iris capture of the intraocular lens.

→ Corneal endothelial damage may be reduced by using preservative-free intracameral solutions and by the addition of glutathione to irrigating solutions.

SELF-ASSESSMENT TEST

1. Name the primary component of most viscoelastics.
2. Advantages of cohesive viscoelastics include (list all that apply)
   a. Ease of removal
   b. Better coating of corneal endothelium
   c. More effective space maintenance
   d. Less likely to "drag" iris or vitreous out of incision
3. Viscoelastics should be completely removed at the close of surgery (list all that apply)
   a. To avoid postoperative intraocular pressure elevation
   b. To prevent endothelial toxicity
   c. To prevent macular edema
   d. To prevent vitreous hemorrhage
4. Corneal endothelium injury during intraocular irrigation may be reduced by (list all that apply)
   a. Directing irrigation port away from endothelium
   b. Limiting use of intraocular antibiotics
   c. Addition of intraocular glutathione
   d. Use of chilled irrigating fluid
5. Name three uses for intraoperative miotics.

For preferred responses to these questions, see pages 223–224.

SUGGESTED READING

Jonas JB, Akkoyun I, Budde WM, Kreissig I, Degenring RF. Intravitreal reinjection of triamcinolone for exudative age-related macular degeneration. *Arch Ophthalmol.* 2004;122:218–222.

Liesegang TJ. Viscoelastic substances in ophthalmology. *Surv Ophthalmol.* 1990;34:268–293.

Pandey SK, Werner L, Escobar-Gomez M, Roig-Melo EA, Apple DJ. Dye-enhanced cataract surgery. Part 1: anterior capsule staining for capsulorrhexis in advanced/white cataract. *J Cataract Refract Surg.* 2000;26:1052–1059.

Parikh CH, Edelhauser HF. Ocular surgical pharmacology: corneal endothelial safety and toxicity. *Curr Opin Ophthalmol.* 2003;14:178–185.

Roth DB, Chieh J, Spirn MJ, Green SN, Yarian DL, Chaudhry NA. Noninfectious endophthalmitis associated with intravitreal triamcinolone injection. *Arch Ophthalmol.* 2003;121:1279–1282.

Chapter 11

Wound Construction in Cataract Surgery

Anthony J. Aldave, MD
Aaleya Koreishi, MD

The surgeon faces many options regarding wound construction, and this chapter discusses the subject of wound construction from the perspective of wound construction in cataract surgery. Cataract surgery, a common type of ophthalmic surgery, is the surgery in which the beginning surgeon is most likely to be involved. Discussion of specific techniques of other types of ophthalmic surgery is beyond the scope of this book.

Although most surgeons now prefer phacoemulsification through a small incision, followed by placement of a foldable or injectable intraocular lens, the need to perform an extracapsular cataract extraction (ECCE) or intracapsular cataract extraction (ICCE) may arise. Therefore, a familiarity with the construction of both small corneal incisions as well as large scleral incisions is important. Decisions encountered when planning cataract surgery include wound location, shape, size, and architecture (scleral tunnel, limbal tunnel or clear corneal).

INSTRUMENTS

The variety of instruments available to construct the cataract surgical wound reflect the varying approaches to the incision (Figure 11.1). The crescent blade is commonly used in the construction of scleral tunnel incisions, first to perform a partial thickness scleral groove, then to carry this incision forward, performing a partial thickness scleral dissection. The keratome is used to enter

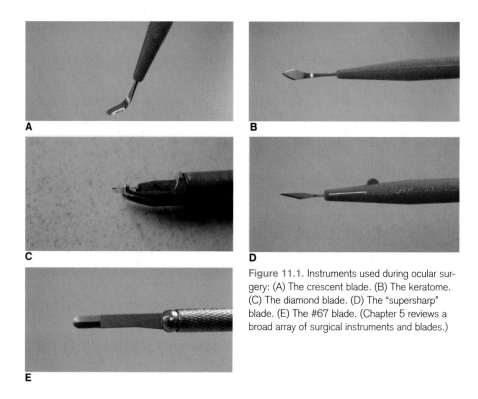

Figure 11.1. Instruments used during ocular surgery: (A) The crescent blade. (B) The keratome. (C) The diamond blade. (D) The "supersharp" blade. (E) The #67 blade. (Chapter 5 reviews a broad array of surgical instruments and blades.)

the anterior chamber. Alternatively, a diamond blade may be used to create the initial scleral incision, the partial thickness scleral dissection, and to enter into the anterior chamber. However, the reduced tissue resistance encountered when using a diamond blade does not provide the tactile feedback that a beginning surgeon uses to become familiar with the feel of a properly constructed wound. When constructing an ECCE incision, the entry into the anterior chamber may be made by a keratome, between 2.7 and 3.2 mm in width, and extended with a crescent blade, a #69 blade, or scissors. Alternatively, a large keratome blade, up to 6 or 7 mm in width, may be used to enlarge the incision, which will need to be expanded to approximately 10 mm to accommodate removal of the intact nucleus.

When performing phacoemulsification cataract extraction, the surgeon may create a scleral tunnel incision using the crescent blade, and enter the anterior chamber entry using a keratome. On the other hand, a clear corneal or limbal incision may be created and the anterior chamber entered with the keratome or diamond blade. A "supersharp" blade may be used to create a paracentesis (side-port stab-incision), through which the phacoemulsification surgeon will inject balanced saline solution, viscoelastics, intraocular anesthetics, and insert second instruments to manipulate the cataractous lens.

LOCATION

The location of the wound is defined by its relation to the limbus and the clock-hour at which it is placed. The surgical limbus consists of two zones, the anterior blue zone over clear cornea, and the posterior white zone over the scleral spur and iris root (Figure 11.2). The conjunctival insertion onto the cornea serves as the anterior boundary of the limbus, whereas the posterior boundary consists of the posterior border of the white zone.

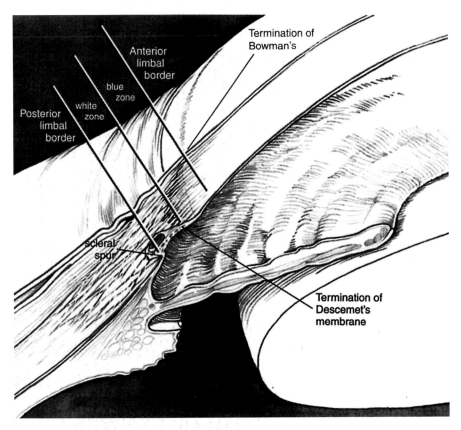

Figure 11.2. Anatomy of the limbus. (Reproduced with permission. From Spaeth GL, ed. *Ophthalmic Surgery Principles and Practice.* 3rd ed. Philadelphia: WB Saunders Co, 2003; 52.)

The mode of cataract removal (extracapsular versus phacoemulsification) dictates where the incision is placed in relation to the limbus. Extracapsular incisions are usually limbal, starting 1 to 2 mm posterior to the anterior limbal border, and scleral tunnel incisions are placed more posteriorly, 2 to 4 mm posterior to the anterior limbal border. Both the distance of an incision from the limbus and the length of an incision may significantly affect the amount of postoperative astigmatism. Typically, the more posterior to the limbus and the shorter the wound length, the less the induced astigmatism (Figure 11.3).

The clock-hour placement of the wound is determined primarily by the surgeon's preferred operating position and comfort. Some right-handed surgeons choose to sit at the head of the bed, and center their incision at the 10 or 11 o'clock position. Others prefer to sit temporally and center the incision at the 7 to 8 o'clock position for a right eye and the 1 to 2 o'clock position for a left eye. The patient's anatomy may also dictate incision location. Specifically, a large nose, deep-set orbit, large brow, corneal opacity, or previous glaucoma procedure may alter the location of the cataract incision.

While most clear corneal cataract incisions are astigmatically neutral, a larger incision, such as an extracapsular cataract incision, tends to affect the corneal curvature in a manner similar to a limbal relaxing incision. The cornea flattens in the meridian of the incision and, through coupling, steepens 90° away. Therefore, the location of the cataract incision may be adjusted based on the patient's preoperative astigmatism, or astigmatic keratectomy may be performed at the time of cataract surgery to address corneal astigmatism.

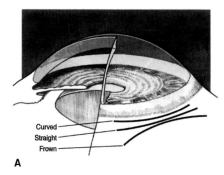

Curved
Straight
Frown

A

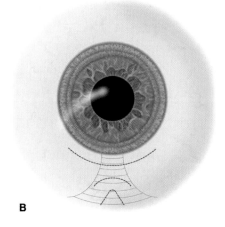

B

Figure 11.3. Koch's incisional funnel. (A) Incisions that fall within a certain size and distance from the limbus are astigmatically neutral. (B) Note how the limbal curvilinear incision is unstable (extends outside the "incisional funnel") but the frown and chevron incisions are stable. (Part A reproduced with permission. From Spaeth GL, ed. *Ophthalmic Surgery Principles and Practice.* 3rd ed. Philadelphia: WB Saunders Co; 2003; 53. Part B illustration by Mark M. Miller.)

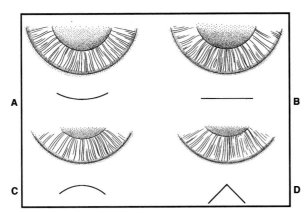

Figure 11.4. Incision shapes. (A) Curvilinear. (B) Straight. (C) Frown. (D) Chevron. (Reproduced with permission. From Masket S. Cataract incision and closure. *Focal Points: Clinical Modules for Ophthalmologists.* San Francisco: American Academy of Ophthalmology; 1995, module 3. Illustration by Christine Gralapp.)

SHAPE

Possible incision shapes include linear, curvilinear (circumferential to the limbus), and frown or chevron-shaped (Figure 11.4). As is true for incision location and length, the shape of the incision affects the induced astigmatic effect, with postoperative astigmatism typically minimized by wounds that curve away from the limbus. Clear corneal incisions are linear as they are created with a planar keratome or diamond blade.

SIZE

The width and length of the incision not only affect the postoperative astigmatism as discussed above, but also play a dynamic role throughout the procedure. The ECCE wound is usually 4 clock hours in length, large enough to deliver the nucleus in one piece. Small-incision cataract surgery using phacoemulsification necessitates a wound size that is large enough to allow the surgeon to manipulate the phaco handpiece and to allow sufficient fluid flow around the handpiece to prevent a thermal wound burn. For either the regular size phaco tip or the microtip, this usually means an incision between 2.7 and 3.2 mm in width. However, the wound should be narrow enough and long enough to prevent excessive egress of viscoelastic and irrigating fluid, maintain a stable anterior chamber, and prevent iris prolapse. For clear corneal cataract incisions, this usually is accomplished with a wound length of at least 2 mm. If the incision is too long (anteroposterior), decreased instrument mobility, excessive corneal striae that interfere with visibility, and difficulty removing sub-incisional cortex result. A small incision may need to be enlarged to accommodate insertion of the intraocular lens, which may be performed with a keratome or #69 blade.

ARCHITECTURE

This section helps the beginning surgeon differentiate extracapsular from phacoemulsification cataract wounds.

Extracapsular Cataract Extraction Wound

The first step in constructing an ECCE wound is a conjunctival peritomy (Figure 11.5A). The conjunctiva and Tenon's membrane are grasped with 0.12 forceps, 2 to 4 mm posterior to the limbus (at the right side of the planned conjunctival peritomy for a right-handed surgeon). Westcott scissors are used to incise the conjunctiva and Tenon's membrane that are tented upwards by the forceps, exposing the underlying bare sclera. The scissors are then used to make a radial incision, dissect the conjunctiva and Tenon's membrane from the globe, and to perform a limbal peritomy for approximately 4 clock hours. When creating the limbal peritomy, the blade of the scissors underneath the conjunctiva is placed against and pushed over the limbus while the forceps are used to retract the cut edge of the conjunctiva posteriorly, leaving no conjunctiva adherent to the limbus as the peritomy is created. Wet-field cautery is then applied for hemostasis.

The first plane of the ECCE incision consists of a groove perpendicular to the scleral surface, of approximately 50% to 60% depth. The groove is placed 1 to 2 mm posterior to the anterior limbal border (this distance can be measured with calipers and marked). A crescent or diamond blade is used to make this incision while the globe is stabilized with 0.12 forceps (Figure 11.5B). A superior rectus bridle suture may be used to aid in globe manipulation. The groove is carried out for the desired length of the curvilinear incision (usually 4 clock hours). The end of the crescent blade is bent to almost 90° and used to create the second plane of the incision (Figure 11.5C). The surgeon moves the blade in a circular motion while maintaining an anterior movement, creating a plane at 50% to 60% scleral thickness to create a partial-thickness sclerectomy. The incision is carried forward into clear cornea. It is important to tilt the crescent blade at the ends of the incision, allowing it to follow the contour of the globe.

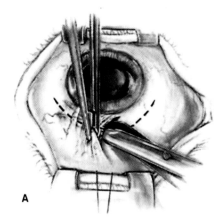

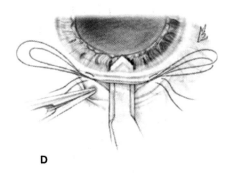

A

D

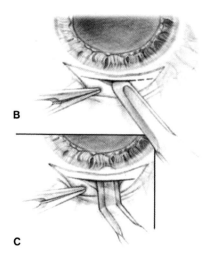

B

C

Figure 11.5. Construction of an extracapsular cataract extraction incision. (A) Conjunctival peritomy. (B) Plane 1: Initial groove perpendicular to the globe. (C) Plane 2: Scleral dissection up to clear cornea. (D) Plane 3: Entry into the anterior chamber. (From Gottsch JD, Stark WJ, Goldberg MF, eds. *Ophthalmic Surgery*. 5th ed. London: Oxford University Press, 1998. Reproduced by permission of Edward Arnold.)

Before making the third plane of the incision, and entering the anterior chamber, a paracentesis is made approximately 2 to 3 clock hours from the center of the ECCE wound, and the surgeon instills viscoelastic to deepen the anterior chamber. The third plane of the incision is made with a keratome, which is maneuvered through the tunnel, up to clear cornea (Figure 11.5D). The heel is lifted as the blade enters the anterior chamber. The surgeon then opens the incision in both directions using a keratome, #69 blade, or scissors. If this large three-plane incision is created successfully, a watertight closure will be possible using only a minimal number of sutures.

Phacoemulsification Cataract Incisions

The three major categories of phacoemulsification cataract wound architecture are scleral tunnel, limbal, and clear corneal incisions. This section introduces you to the specific indications, advantages, and disadvantages of each category.

Scleral Tunnel Incision

Phacoemulsification allows for small incision cataract surgery. As the surgeon who is learning phacoemulsification wound construction will typically need to suture the incision closed, the location of the incision posterior to the limbus results in less suture-induced astigmatism, and the risk of a thermal corneal burn is significantly decreased. Additionally, if the integrity of the posterior capsule is compromised during the procedure, the scleral tunnel incision may be easily converted to an extracapsular cataract incision. Therefore, it is imperative that the beginning phaco surgeon become facile with the construction of scleral tunnel incisions prior to performing clear corneal incisional surgery.

The initial step in creation of the scleral tunnel incision is the creation of a limbal peritomy (as previously described). The anterior chamber is filled with viscoelastic material injected through a paracentesis created approximately 3 to 4 clock hours from the main incision.

After cautery is used to obtain adequate hemostasis, toothed forceps are used to secure the globe as the initial scleral incision is made with a blade held perpendicular to the globe. This incision is created at a depth of 50% to 60% scleral thickness, 2 to 4 millimeters posterior to the limbus (Figure 11.6A). A crescent blade is then used to perform a lamellar scleral dissection anteriorly to clear cornea (Figure11.6B). It is very important to maintain a constant depth: if the end of the crescent blade is angled too far anteriorly (toe up, heel down), the roof of the tunnel, and wound integrity, will be compromised; if the end of the blade is pointed too far posteriorly (toe down, heel up), premature entry into the globe is possible with resultant iris prolapse.

The third plane of the incision is made with a keratome or diamond blade. The blade is advanced to the anterior extent of the scleral tunnel until it is visualized in clear cornea. The heel of the blade is then lifted off of the sclera as the tip faces into the anterior chamber. With controlled forward pressure, the blade is allowed to enter the anterior chamber, completing the triplanar incision (Figure 11.6C).

Limbal Incision

The limbal incision has benefits over the scleral tunnel incision. It tends to be easier and take less time to construct. Possible advantages over the clear

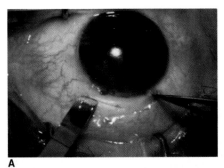

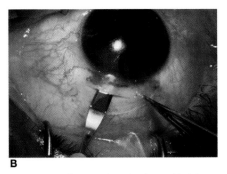

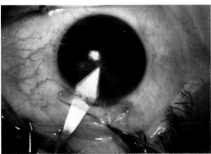

Figure 11.6. Creating the scleral tunnel incision. (A) Initial groove created using a crescent blade. (B) Dissecting through partial-thickness sclera up to clear cornea. (C) Anterior chamber entry with a keratome. (Reproduced with permission. From Jones DT, Karp CL, Heigle TJ: Principles and techniques of cataract surgery phacoemulsification: methodology and complications. In: Albert DM, ed. *Ophthalmic Surgery: Principles and Techniques*. Boston: Blackwell Science: 1999:283–312.)

corneal incision are (1) faster healing due to the proximity of the conjunctival vessels, (2) more rapid postoperative stabilization, and (3) less induced astigmatism. However, the risk of developing conjunctival chemosis, which may interfere with insertion of instruments into the incision and visibility of the anterior chamber secondary to pooling of fluid on the cornea, is greater than with clear corneal incisions. A two-plane posterior limbal incision, located 1 to 2 mm posterior to the anterior limbal border, has been touted to be superior to the clear corneal wound in terms of stability.

Clear Corneal Incision

Construction of the clear corneal incision is the most efficient in terms of instruments and time required for its creation. Only topical anesthesia is required, obviating the need for patient sedation during the administration of a peribulbar or retrobulbar block (see Chapter 9), eliminating the risk of globe perforation associated with needle placement in the orbit, and allowing patients to continue anticoagulation therapy. Additionally, as a conjunctival peritomy is not required, the incision does not interfere with previous or subsequent glaucoma surgery nor is it affected by scarring or thinning of the conjunctiva or sclera. The technique of creating a three-plane clear corneal incision involves making an initial groove (half corneal thickness) using a crescent blade or diamond blade. A keratome or the diamond blade is then used to dissect a lamellar corneal tunnel approximately 2 mm in length. The third plane of the incision is made as the heel of the blade is lifted off the cornea, and the point is directed into the anterior chamber (Figure 11.7).

Although the clear corneal incision takes the least time to create and, if created properly, is self-sealing (not requiring suture closure), it is associated with several potential disadvantages and complications. Inadequate construction may result in the intraoperative difficulties previously mentioned. Additionally, if compromise of posterior capsular integrity occurs intraoperatively, the surgeon may need to close a temporal clear corneal incision and move superiorly to create an extracapsular cataract incision. Several postoperative complications may develop following cataract surgery through a clear corneal incision. A corneal thermal injury (phaco burn) is often not amenable to closure with sutures or tissue adhesive and may require placement of a corneal

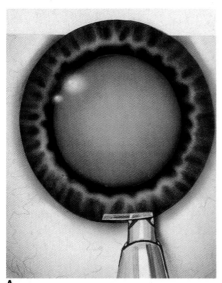

A

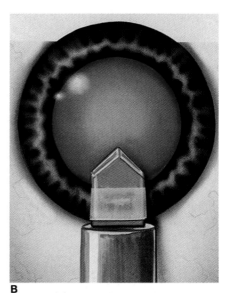

B

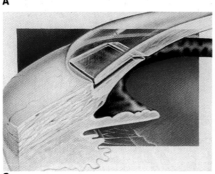

C

Figure 11.7. Three-planed clear corneal incision made with a diamond blade. (A and B) Surgeon's view. (C) Cross-sectional view. (Reproduced with permission. From Burratto L, ed. *Phacoemulsification Principles and Techniques.* Thorofare, NJ: Slack Inc, 1998;6.)

patch graft for closure. Iris prolapse into a temporal clear corneal incision during surgery may result in iris atrophy with postoperative polycoria and photophobia. Several recent reports have noted an increased rate of endophthalmitis associated with clear corneal incisions when compared with scleral tunnel incisions, prompting some cataract surgeons to routinely place a suture in all clear corneal incisions.

KEY POINTS

→ The crescent knife, keratome, diamond knife, and various other microsurgical blades are used to create incisions.

→ Incisions may be multiplanar or uniplanar and include anterior limbal (for extracapsular surgery), posterior limbal, scleral tunnel, and clear corneal locations (for phacoemulsification surgery).

→ Larger and more anterior incisions usually result in greater astigmatism.

→ Incisions must be large enough to allow cataract extraction and IOL insertion; too-large wounds result in increased postoperative astigmatism and less intraoperative control of anterior chamber depth due to excess fluid egress.

→ Clear corneal incisions require only topical anesthesia, do not interfere with previous conjunctival surgery (as in previous trabeculectomy surgery), require little time to create, and may not require suture closure.

SELF-ASSESSMENT TEST

1. Induced postoperative astigmatism increases with
   a. More anterior limbal incision
   b. Longer length of incision
   c. Wounds curving away from limbus
   d. All of the above
2. Name two intraperative problems created by an incision that is too wide.
3. Name the three planes of the standard extracapsular cataract incision.
4. List two possible disadvantages of clear corneal incisions.

For preferred responses to these questions, see pages 223–224.

SUGGESTED READING

Ellis MF. Topical anaesthesia: a risk factor for post-cataract extraction endophthalmitis. *Clin Experiment Ophthalmol.* 2003;31:125–128.

Ernest P, Tipperman R, Eagle R, et al. Is there a difference in incision healing based on location? *J Cataract Refract Surg.* 1998;24:482–486.

Ernest PH, Neuhann T. Posterior limbal incision. *J Cataract Refract Surg.* 1996;22:78–84.

Koch PS. Structural analysis of cataract incision construction. *J Cataract Refract Surg.* 1991;17:661–667.

Lertsumitkul S, Myers PC, O'Rourke MT, Chandra J. Endophthalmitis in the western Sydney region: a case-control study. *Clin Experiment Ophthalmol.* 2001;29:400–405.

Lyle WA, Jin GJ. Prospective evaluation of early visual and refractive effects with small clear corneal incision for cataract surgery. *J Cataract Refract Surg.* 1996;22:1456–1460.

Nagaki Y, Hayasaka S, Kadoi C, et al. Bacterial endophthalmitis after small incision cataract surgery. Effect of incision placement and intraocular lens type. *J Cataract Refract Surg.* 2003;29:20–26.

Norregaard JC, Thoning H, Bernth-Petersen P, Andersen TF, Javitt JC, Anderson GF. Risk of endophthalmitis after cataract extraction: results from the International Cataract Surgery Outcomes Study. *Br J Ophthalmol.* 1997;81:102–106.

Pallin SL. Chevron sutureless closure: a preliminary report. *J Cataract Refract Surg.* 1991;17:706–709.

Pfleger T, Skorpik C, Menapace R, et al. Long-term course of induced astigmatism after clear corneal incision cataract surgery. *J Cataract Refract Surg.* 1996;22:72–77.

Singer JA. Frown incision for minimizing induced astigmatism after small incision cataract surgery with rigid optic intraocular lens implantation. *J Cataract Refract Surg.* 1991;17:677–688.

Chapter 12

Suturing and Knot Tying

Edward J. Wladis, MD
Paul D. Langer, MD

Optimal wound closure apposes the separate edges of the wound, thereby providing critical physical support to the tissue during the early phases of healing. Meticulous surgical technique and proper knot tying enable the clinician to achieve the functional aspects of wound closure without distortion of the tissue.

This chapter describes techniques of simple wound closure, starting with placement of a square surgical knot; reviews basic principles for needle handling in suture placement; and covers techniques for placement of interrupted, continuous, and mattress sutures. (See Chapter 6 for the overview of surgical instrumentation and materials, including suture characteristics and sutures commonly used in ophthalmic surgery.)

SIMPLE SQUARE KNOT (INSTRUMENT TIE)

Tying a square knot is a basic skill in suturing; success in placing more complex sutures largely depends upon mastering this technique. Placing a square knot involves the following steps.

1. The needle is passed through both sides of the wound and pulled until the opposite end is sufficiently short (Figure 12.1A). At that point, the needle is released, and forceps are used to grasp the long end of the suture approximately 3 cm from the wound. The needle holder is then held in the center of the wound just to the right of the suture (for a right-handed surgeon) with the jaws closed and pointing away from the surgeon (Figure 12.1B). The first loop of the knot is then wrapped around the tip of the waiting needle holder (Figure 12.1C).

2. A second and even third loop can be wrapped around the needle holder, depending on the tension of the wound and size of the suture, in order to prevent the wound from gaping after the first loops are tied down. (For example, three loops may be required for 10-0 nylon sutures in the cornea, but only one loop is necessary for skin closure in the eyelids.) The jaws of the needle holder are then opened and the opposite, short end of the suture is grasped (Figure 12.1D).

3. The short end of the suture is pulled towards the surgeon, and the long end away from the surgeon, with sufficient tension to approximate the walls of the wound with only slight eversion (Figure 12.1E). Care should be taken to avoid excessive tension, as this may result in excessive tissue eversion after healing or in strangulation of the tissue with subsequent ischemia and tissue necrosis. When one or more loops are tied down, it is referred to as a *throw*.

4. At this point, the surgeon releases the end of the suture held by the needle holder and repositions the closed needle holder in the center of the wound, again to the right of the suture (for a right-handed surgeon), but now pointing toward the surgeon and the short end of the suture. The long end of the suture is then looped over the closed tips of the needle holder (Figure 12.1F).

5. Again, the jaws of the forceps are opened and the short end of the suture is grasped; however, this time the short end of the suture grasped by the needle holder is pulled *away* from the surgeon while the longer suture end grasped by the forceps is pulled *toward* the surgeon, tightening the knot (Figure 12.1G).

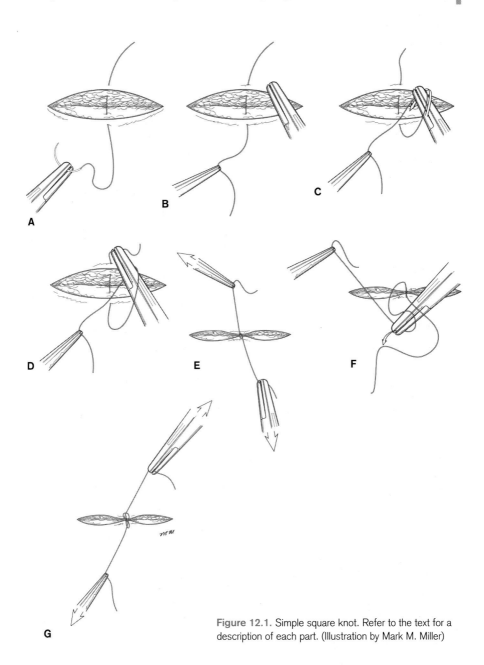

A

B

C

D

E

F

G

Figure 12.1. Simple square knot. Refer to the text for a description of each part. (Illustration by Mark M. Miller)

The result of this sequence, in which two throws are tied down in opposite directions, is one *square knot.* When the first throw of a knot consists of two loops, the result is termed a *surgeon's knot;* this technique is used when the wound tension would cause the first throw of a square knot to loosen. In ophthalmology it is customary to place *three* loops in the first throw of the knot when using 10-0 nylon because of the tendency for 10-0 suture to loosen.

Typically, one additional throw is placed over a square knot or a surgeon's knot to complete the tie, although in some circumstances, two knots (four throws) or more can be placed if unraveling of the knot is a concern. Regardless of the number of knots placed, it is critical that each consecutive throw result in the two ends of the suture each being pulled from one side of the wound to the opposite side; only in this fashion will the knot be "square."

BASIC SUTURING PRINCIPLES

When placing sutures, the surgeon grasps the needle near the tip of the needle holder, at a point on the needle approximately two-thirds the distance from the needle tip to the swaged end (where the suture is attached). The needle should enter the tissue *perpendicular to the tip of the needle* (Figure 12.2); such positioning frequently requires slight pronation of the wrist. In the case of a highly curved (such as a half-circle) needle, considerable wrist pronation may be necessary. The needle is then passed through the tissue by gently rotating the wrist in a motion that allows the suture to "follow the curvature of the needle" and slide easily through the tissue; the needle should not be "pushed" or forced through the tissue. At the same time, the edge of the wound where the needle is to be passed is grasped with forceps in the non-dominant hand; the tissue in the forceps is not released until the needle is re-grasped with the needle holder after the needle emerges from the wound. The forceps should not grasp the needle as it emerges from the wound, as this will dull the needle unnecessarily.

While the underlying principles governing suture placement are identical for all procedures, the requirements of specific types of surgery deserve special mention.

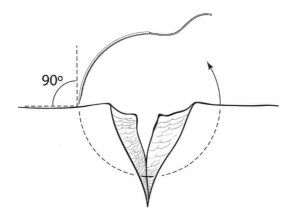

Figure 12.2. Position of entry for a highly curved needle. (Illustration by Mark M. Miller)

Corneal Suturing

In cases requiring corneal suturing (as in penetrating keratoplasty), fine forceps (Castroviejo 0.12 mm forceps, Figure 5.24) should be used to firmly grasp the tissue but without damaging it. The 10-0 suture can then be driven beneath the forceps. Optimal technique requires radial placement of the needle in the case of a penetrating keratoplasty, or placement perpendicular to the wound when repairing corneal lacerations.

The tension on the corneal sutures determines the ultimate astigmatism found in corneal transplants and in repair of lacerations. As a result, these procedures require technique that creates enough suture tension necessary for sufficient closure but that avoids excess tension, which leads to significant astigmatism. Thus, sutures should be tied in a fashion that closes the wound with uniform tension but does not create lines of tension on the graft (or in a lacerated cornea). All suture sites should be checked with fluorescein (ie, Seidel) testing to be sure that there is no leakage from the wound.

Suturing in Strabismus Surgery

In strabismus surgery, the goal is to suture a surgically detached muscle back to the underlying sclera. Special care must be taken in these cases to avoid needle penetration of the sclera, which in turn might lead to a retinal hole. The potential for this serious complication is minimized by the use of a spatula needle. A spatula needle is flat on its underside and sharp on its outer edges;

this design promotes a needle pass that maintains a steady depth during its passage through tissue, since the bottom surface of the needle is smooth. The needle is passed carefully through the sclera with attention directed to a "flat" needle approach and constant needle depth.

COMMON SUTURING TECHNIQUES

In ophthalmology, several types of sutures are commonly used in wound closure:

→ Simple interrupted suture: basic tool
→ Vertical mattress suture: greater support
→ Near–far vertical mattress suture: raising subcutaneous tissue
→ Horizontal mattress suture: minimizing tension
→ Simple continuous (running) suture: rapid closure
→ Running horizontal mattress suture: speed and tension dispersion
→ Buried interrupted subcutaneous suture: minimizing closure tension subcutaneously
→ Running subcuticular suture: closing the skin without penetrating the epidermis

Simple Interrupted Suture

The interrupted suture is the basic tool of wound closure. To place an interrupted suture, the surgeon drives the needle from one edge of the wound through the underlying deep tissue, across the wound, and then through and out the tissue at the opposite side of the wound. Care should be taken to pass the needle at equal depths on both sides of the wound and equidistant from both sides of the wound edge (Figure 12.3). The needle can be passed across the wound in one bite or, if the pass is difficult, the needle can be re-grasped after passing through the initial side of the wound and passed through the opposite side of the wound in a second bite. Square knots are then placed and the ends of the suture are cut; when wound closure is complete, the knots are rotated to the same side of the wound.

Enough interrupted sutures are placed to create adequate strength for secure wound closure. Generally, the first suture is placed in the center of the wound, and each subsequent suture splits the remaining open portion of the wound in half until closure is achieved.

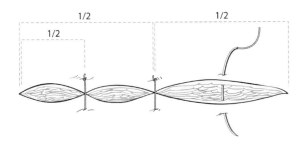

Figure 12.3. Simple inter-rupted suture. (Illustration by Mark M. Miller)

Vertical Mattress Suture

When greater support is needed to close a wound, vertical mattress sutures may be employed (Figure 12.4). The needle should be inserted a short distance from the wound edge and driven across the subcutaneous tissue, exiting on the contralateral side at a distance that is equidistant to that of the insertion. A wider site of needle insertion creates greater tension. The surgeon should then reload the needle so that it faces the opposite direction and the needle should be inserted on the side from which it just exited. However, the insertion should now be more distal to the wound edge than the previous site of exit. The surgeon then drives the needle through the wound so that it exits farther from the wound edge on the initial side than the initial entry point. The dis-tance between the two suture penetrations on each side of the wound should be identical. The suture ends are then tied on the same side of the wound.

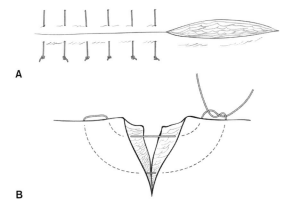

Figure 12.4. (A) Vertical mat-tress sutures may be used to close a wound when greater support is needed. (B) The suture ends are tied on the same side of the wound. (Illus-tration by Mark M. Miller)

Figure 12.5. Near–far vertical mattress suture. (Illustration by Mark M. Miller)

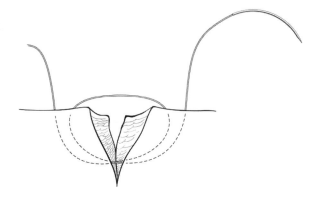

The vertical mattress suture has a strong tendency to evert wound edges, so care should be taken not to over tighten the knots, in order to avoid excess eversion and a poorly healing wound. In ophthalmology, the vertical mattress suture is most frequently used when closing a lacerated (or incised) eyelid margin, where it provides strength as well as an everting tendency, preventing an eyelid margin "notch."

Near–Far Vertical Mattress Suture

In cases where one wishes to raise the subcutaneous tissue, the near–far mattress suture is a useful variation (Figure 12.5). The technique is largely the same as the standard vertical mattress, but the needle initially is driven proximal to the wound and exits distal to the edge on the contralateral side. It then enters on the second side near the wound edge and exits on the initial side far from the wound edge, in a "figure eight" pattern.

Horizontal Mattress Suture

The horizontal mattress suture is largely used to minimize wound tension by displacing tension away from the wound edge (Figure 12.6). To place a horizontal mattress suture, the surgeon enters on one side of the wound, drives the needle across the underlying tissue, and exits on the opposite side of the wound equidistant from the insertion. The surgeon then re-enters on the second side laterally, again equidistant from the wound edge, and drives the needle back through and out the first side, creating a "rectangle" out of the suture. The ends of the suture are then tied on the same side of the wound.

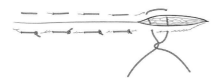

Figure 12.6. Horizontal mattress suture. (Illustration by Mark M. Miller)

In ophthalmology, horizontal mattress sutures are frequently used when tying bolsters across the upper and lower eyelids to close the palpebral aperture temporarily. They are also sometimes employed to close scleral tunnel incisions after cataract surgery.

Simple Continuous (Running) Suture

Running sutures permit the surgeon to close wounds much more rapidly than other techniques (Figure 12.7A). Essentially, a simple suture is placed in the same fashion as an interrupted suture at one end of the wound, but in the case of running sutures, the thread attached to the needle is not cut. The surgeon places another simple suture by returning to the initial side and driving the needle to the contralateral side. No knot is tied until the surgeon reaches the termination of the length of the wound. A single knot is then placed, using the last loop tied as a suture end. Alternatively, in order to avoid distorting

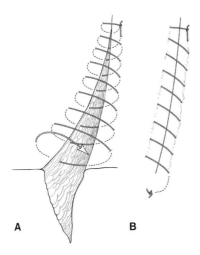

Figure 12.7. (A) Simple continuous (running) suture. (B) Alternate final knot. (Illustration by Mark M. Miller)

A   B

the end of the wound, a final bite can be taken in tissue just outside the end of the wound and this loop tied as a suture end (Figure 12.7B). Proper technique necessitates evenly spaced bites and the adjustment of suture tension prior to tying the final knot to ensure an even distribution of wound tension.

While running sutures save time (as well as suture), they have a greater tendency to strangulate or pucker the wound edges. Furthermore, any break along the string (or in a knot) can weaken the entire closure, whereas in an interrupted closure only a localized weakness would develop after a break.

Running Horizontal Mattress Suture

The horizontal mattress suture affords the surgeon the benefits of speed and dispersion of tension (Figure 12.8). The surgeon enters on one side of the wound, passes the needle through the underlying deep tissue, and exits on the contralateral side equidistant from the point of insertion. The suture is then passed laterally on the second side before passage back across the subcutaneous tissue to the first side. This process is then repeated until the surgeon reaches the end of the wound, and a knot is then tied to the final suture loop.

Buried Interrupted Subcutaneous Suture

In many cases, subcutaneous sutures are needed to minimize the tension of closure (Figure 12.9). To place a subcutaneous suture such that the knot is

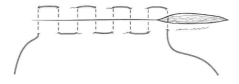

Figure 12.8. Running horizontal mattress suture. (Illustration by Mark M. Miller)

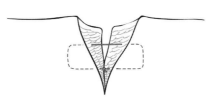

Figure 12.9. Buried interrupted subcutaneous suture. (Illustration by Mark M. Miller)

buried, the surgeon should evert the wound edge mildly, and should enter the wound in the dermis as close to the base as possible. The needle is then passed to exit through the dermis superiorly on the same side, and is passed through the superior dermal edge of the contralateral side, at a depth equal to the depth where the needle emerged from the initial side. The suture should then travel to the base of the wound, where it should exit at a depth equal to the depth of the initial needle entry. When the knot is tied, it will lie deep to the tissue closed by the suture.

Running Subcuticular Suture

A skin incision can be closed without penetrating the epidermis across the wound by means of a running subcuticular suture. The advantage of such a suture is a less conspicuous scar.

A running subcuticular suture is placed by first entering the skin at a point outside the termination of a wound and perpendicular to it, passing the needle toward the wound edge. The needle emerges just under the skin from one side of the wound. The needle then enters the opposite side of the wound, just below the skin at the edge of the wound, is passed subcutaneously parallel to the skin surface, and exits just below the skin edge (Figure 12.10A). The needle is then placed in the opposite (first) side of the wound, just below the skin, at a point directly opposite where the needle just exited. A subcutaneous

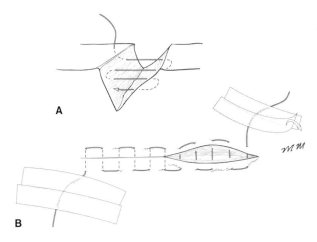

Figure 12.10. Running subcuticular suture. (A) Subcutaneous bites parallel to the skin surface. (B) Ends affixed with steri-strips. (Illustration by Mark M. Miller)

bite of identical length is then taken, parallel to the skin surface, again exiting just below the skin. In this fashion, successive bites are taken on alternate sides of the wound, always just beneath the skin, with the bites "staggered" on each side by a distance of one length of a "bite."

At the completion of the wound closure, the final needle bite on one side should be passed subcutaneously through the wound on the opposite side and then out onto the skin. The two ends of the suture are not tied but simply affixed to the skin with steri-strips (Figure 12.10B). The suture is pulled out of the wound from one end 5 to 7 days after placement.

KEY POINTS

→ Proper suture technique supports incisional edges during the early healing phases to facilitate more rapid healing with less scarring.

→ The square knot may be placed with additional loops in the first throw (surgeon's knot) to allow stability against wound tension and the tendency of microscopic suture to slip with only one loop.

→ Correct suturing technique includes avoiding grasp of the needle tip, entering tissue perpendicular, and following the curve of the needle.

→ Excessive suture tension may result in wound edge eversion, tissue strangulation, and, for corneoscleral incisions, increased astigmatism.

SELF-ASSESSMENT TEST

1. The surgeon places two loops in the first throw of a surgical knot (list all that apply)
   a. Always
   b. To prevent loosening of the knot while tying
   c. Only in mattress sutures
   d. In a "surgeon's knot"
2. During suturing (list all that apply)
   a. The needle is grasped at its blunt end to avoid damaging the tip.
   b. The needle should enter the tissue perpendicular to the tip of the needle.
   c. The surgeon should follow the curvature of the needle in passing the suture.
   d. As the needle emerges from the tissue, it should be grasped at its tip to avoid tissue damage.

3. Excess tension on a corneal suture (list all that apply)
   a. May produce astigmatism
   b. May induce wound leakage
   c. May be avoided by placing the suture in a radial fashion
   d. Does not occur with 10-0 nylon
4. The continuous suture technique (list all that apply)
   a. Requires less time than interrupted sutures
   b. May produce greater wound dehiscence than interrupted sutures if the suture breaks
   c. Is reserved for subcuticular closures
   d. May produce uneven wound tension and "puckering"
   e. Requires more suture material than interrupted suture technique

For preferred responses to these questions, see pages 223–224.

SUGGESTED READING

Ethicon. *Knot Tying Manual*. Somerville, NJ: Ethicon; 2005.

Dunn DL, cont ed. *Wound Closure Manual*. Somerville, NJ: Ethicon; undated.

Chapter 13

Hemostasis

J. Paul Dieckert, MD

Hemostasis in ocular surgery is vital to achieving surgical objectives, visualizing important structures, increasing operative safety, and minimizing surgical complications. This chapter organizes the subject into six key areas: prevention, heating, vasoconstriction, biochemical enhancement of hemostasis, mechanical tamponade, and embolization.

PREVENTION

In ophthalmic plastic surgery, preoperative control of hypertension and avoidance of aspirin 2 weeks prior to surgery are important measures to diminish risk of excessive intraoperative and postoperative bleeding. The reverse Trendelenburg position reduces venous congestion and may lessen the risk of hemorrhage associated with anesthetic injection. Hypotensive anesthesia can be an important intraoperative preventative measure. In patients with classic hemophilia, intravenous (IV) cryoprecipitated factor VIII has been used effectively to prevent hemorrhage during retrobulbar anesthesia and peripheral iridectomy in patients with classic hemophilia. As citric acid in balanced salt solution causes a 50% increase in bleeding times, avoidance of irrigating solutions containing citric acid is recommended in trauma and other cases prone to heavy bleeding.

HEATING

The use of heat to achieve hemostasis is achieved by cautery, diathermy, and photocoagulation.

Cautery

Cautery, once common in eyelid procedures, involves the application of an electrically heated wire to bleeding vessels. The heating induces coagulation of tissue proteins. The coagulum then acts as a barrier to further blood flow, followed by blanching, charring, and tissue contraction.

Diathermy

Diathermy, either monopolar or bipolar, achieves heating by passing an electric current through the target tissue (Figures 13.1, 13.2, and 13.3). The resistance of the tissue to the electrical current results in heating of the tissue with subsequent coagulation of proteins and the formation of a coagulum that prevents further blood flow. Bipolar diathermy is preferred because it restricts the current to an elliptical field between two electrodes and avoids passage of current with inadvertent heating injury to nontarget tissues. Diathermy requires direct visualization of the bleeding vessel and is difficult to achieve if diffuse bleeding is present. Excessive diathermy leads to tissue destruction and necrosis. Multifunction instruments with combined bipolar diathermy, aspiration, and reflux are useful in controlling intraocular bleeding during vitrectomy by minimiz-

Figure 13.1. Bipolar diathermy forceps.

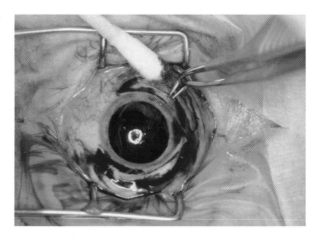

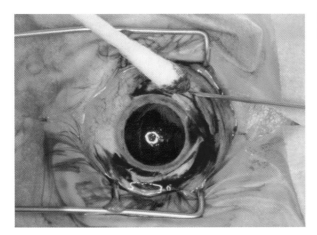

Figure 13.2. Bipolar diathermy probe.

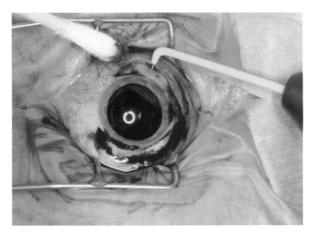

Figure 13.3. Monopolar diathermy probe.

ing the need for multiple instrument exchange. Bipolar diathermy instruments with a tapered blunt tip and 23-gauge diameter are useful in trabeculectomy.

Laser Photocoagulation

Laser photocoagulation achieves heating by application of laser energy to the target tissue. Absorption of the laser energy by the target tissue results in localized heating that creates a coagulum and a secondary barrier to blood flow. Endophotocoagulation is applied via a handheld intraocular probe. The probe contains a fiberoptic line that directly carries the laser energy from a diode or argon laser to the intraocular target tissue. Laser photocoagulation does not require direct contact with bleeding tissue. By aspirating blood, raising intraocular pressure, and applying photocoagulation to the hemoglobin within the bleeding vessels, hemostasis can be achieved. The carbon dioxide laser has been found to be useful in orbital surgery for hemostasis. The carbon dioxide laser has been used effectively to prevent bleeding during excision of lymphangiomatous tissue involving the ocular adnexa by flash boiling intracellular water at extremely high temperature and creating a thin layer of heat-coagulated tissue in which blood vessels smaller than 1 mm are sealed.

VASOCONSTRICTION

Vasoconstriction is achieved through the application of epinephrine to the target tissue. The vasoconstriction induced by the epinephrine diminishes blood flow and allows hemostasis to occur. Epinephrine-induced vasoconstriction is restricted to extraocular adnexal surgery in the eyelids and orbit and is available in a premixed proprietary preparation of lidocaine and epinephrine diluted by 1:100000 for use in local infiltrative anesthesia. Epinephrine is also added to intraocular irrigating solutions primarily to maintain mydriasis.

BIOCHEMICAL ENHANCEMENT OF HEMOSTASIS

Thrombin is the mainstay of biochemical enhancement of hemostasis. It can be used in both intra- and extraocular surgery. Thrombin converts fibrinogen to fibrin, induces platelet aggregation, and is nontoxic to the corneal endothelium. It can be used topically or intraocularly. Gelfoam soaked with thrombin and used as a stent in dacryocystorhinostomy is useful for hemostasis and does not have to be removed.

Intraocular thrombin is very useful in treatment of penetrating ocular injuries. Thrombin at 100 units/ml is infused intraocularly via the infusion line when bleeding is encountered. In diabetic patients, thrombin can cause excessive postoperative inflammation and sometimes sterile hypopyon in diabetic patients.

Surgeons using thrombin intraoperatively should be aware of the dangers of inadvertent intravenous administration. Many surgeons are unaware of the potentially lethal effect of inadvertent IV injection of thrombin. Wesley reported rapid death in an animal model using a dosage similar to that used in ocular surgery. Care should be taken to label or color code containers containing thrombin to avoid accidental IV injection. Heparin injection prior to and after thrombin injection has been shown to prevent the lethal effect in an animal model.

MECHANICAL TAMPONADE

Mechanical tamponade refers to the direct application of physical force to staunch blood flow from a bleeding vessel. Raising intraocular pressure is the most common and effective way to mechanically control intraocular bleeding. Increased intraocular pressure is translated into increased transmural pressure of the blood vessel wall that causes collapse or slowing down of blood flow. This is readily accomplished be raising the level of the infusion bottle. Elevating the intraocular pressure risks ocular ischemia and stress to surgical repair of surgical wounds.

Fluid–gas exchange mechanically achieves hemostasis by elevating intraocular pressure via control of pump pressure. Intraocular gas has a higher surface tension than intraocular saline and impedes blood flow. Fluid trapped behind a gas bubble has higher concentration of coagulation factors, which contributes to hemostasis. Intraocular gases unfortunately can impede visibility during surgery, and this technique is usually reserved for the last minutes of the operation.

Other intraocular substances can help control intraoperative bleeding. Perfluorooctane may control intraocular bleeding during vitreoretinal surgery by direct compression or concentration of clotting factors near the bleeding site. Silicone oil controls bleeding by two mechanisms: first, by physical compression and second by concentrating clotting factors in a smaller space. Silicone oil interferes with other intraocular maneuvers and is used typically at the end of surgery. Sodium hyaluronate mechanically confines blood and enhances visualization. It unfortunately also has mild antiplatelet and anticoagulation properties.

Gelfoam (absorbable gelatin sponge), Surgicel (oxidized regenerated cellulose), and Avitene (microfibrillar collagen) are useful mechanical measures to control and confine intraoperative bleeding in ocular adnexal surgery.

Wound closure is a straightforward technique of mechanically controlling intraoperative bleeding. Direct compression to bleeding vortex veins is useful in strabismus and retinal surgery where vortex vein injury can occur.

EMBOLIZATION

Preoperative arteriography and embolization with polyvinyl alcohol foam, metrizamide dissolved in dimethyl sulfoxide, steel coils, gel foam particles, and n–butyl cyanoacrylate has been reported to be useful preoperatively in minimizing hemorrhage during excision of orbital lymphangiomas and arteriovenous malformations. Inadvertent unintended injury to the optic nerve and retina and spasm of the ophthalmic artery may occur during embolization therapy.

KEY POINTS

→ The ophthalmic surgeon has a wide array of preventative, mechanical, and pharmacologic techniques to control surgical bleeding.

→ The experienced surgeon applies appropriate measures in a timely fashion to enhance surgical results and surgical efficiency in ophthalmic surgery.

SELF-ASSESSMENT TEST

1. Measures to prevent excessive bleeding include (list all that apply)
   a. Discontinuance of aspirin
   b. Avoidance of nitric oxide in irrigating fluids
   c. Hypotensive anesthesia
   d. Control of hypertension
2. The major advantage of bipolar diathermy is
   a. Focus of heating energy on target area
   b. Lack of coagulum production
   c. Increased tissue destruction
   d. Simultaneous tamponade
3. Epinephrine (list all that apply)
   a. May be used in intraocular solutions
   b. Shortens duration of infiltrative anesthesia
   c. Reduces bleeding by its biochemical enhancement of hemostasis
   d. Is a potent vasoconstrictor
4. Name two risks of use of thrombin for hemostasis.
5. Name two methods of creating tamponade in intraocular surgery.

For preferred responses to these questions, see pages 223–224.

SUGGESTED READING

de Bustros S. Intraoperative control of hemorrhage in penetrating ocular injuries. *Retina*. 1990;10S:55–58.

Fleischman J, Lerner BC, Reimels H. A new intraocular aspiration probe with bipolar cautery and reflux capabilities. *Arch Ophthalmol*. 1989;107:283.

Jordan DR, Anderson RL. Carbon dioxide laser therapy for conjunctival lymphangioma. *Ophthalmic Surg*. 1987;18:728–730.

Kim SH, Cho YS, Choi YJ. Intraocular hemocoagulase in human vitrectomy. *Jpn J Ophthalmol*. 1994;38:49–55.

Leone CR Jr. Gelfoam-thrombin dacryocystorhinostomy stent. *Am J Ophthalmol*. 1982;94:412–413.

Mannis MJ, Sweet E, Landers MB, et al. Uses of thrombin in ocular surgery. *Arch Ophthalmol*. 1988;106:251–253.

Maxwell DP Jr, Orlick ME, Diamond JG. Intermittent intraocular thrombin as an adjunct to vitrectomy. *Ophthalmic Surg*. 1989;20:108–111.

Rothkoff L, Biedner B, Shoham K. Bilateral cataract extraction in classic haemophilia with retrobulbar anaesthesia and peripheral iridectomy. *Br J Ophthalmol*. 1977;61:765–766.

Shields BM. Evaluation of a tapered, blunt, bipolar cautery tip for trabeculectomy. *Ophthalmic Surg*. 1994;25:54–56.

Verdoorn C, Hendrikse F. Intraocular human thrombin infusion in diabetic vitrectomies. *Ophthalmic Surg*. 1989;20:278–279.

Wesley JR, Wesley RE. A study of the lethal effects of intravenous injection of thrombin in rabbits. *Ann Ophthalmol*. 1990;22:457–459.

Wesley RE. *Techniques in Ophthalmic Plastic Surgery*. New York: John Wiley & Sons, 1986;231.

Part IV

Postoperative Considerations

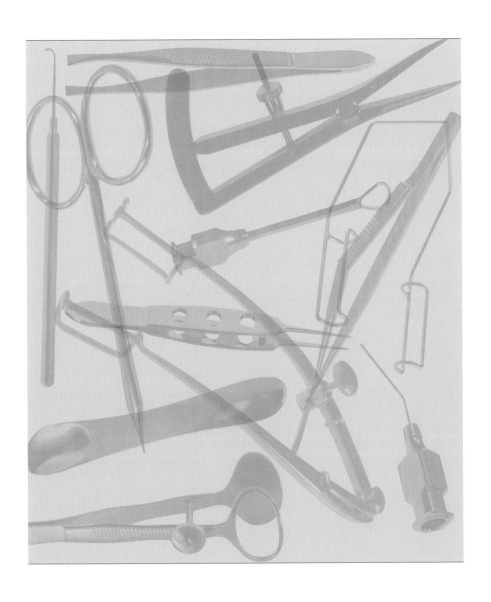

Chapter 14

The Healing Process

Frank Moya, MD
Peter Quiros, MD
Casey Mickler, MS
Oscar A. Cruz, MD

Healing in ophthalmic surgery involves several tissues with differing characteristics. Although many features are common to all tissue types, the processes involved in healing vary accordingly. Wound modulation and healing in the next 5 to 10 years will be much more complex. The manipulation of growth factors, cytokines, and cellular messengers that were once thought only basic science research likely will be indispensable in the operating room and outpatient settings. This chapter addresses the stages and factors involved in healing and the ways in which they impact ocular surgery. An introduction to the basic science of wound modulation will place the surgeon in good stead to improve surgical outcomes in the coming years.

HEALING BY INTENTION

Traditionally, three types of wound healing are described: healing by first intention, second intention, or third intention (Figure 14.1 typifies the first two categories).

First Intention

Healing through first intention involves approximation of the wound edges with sutures or adhesive strips, usually after surgical incision. Wounds healed

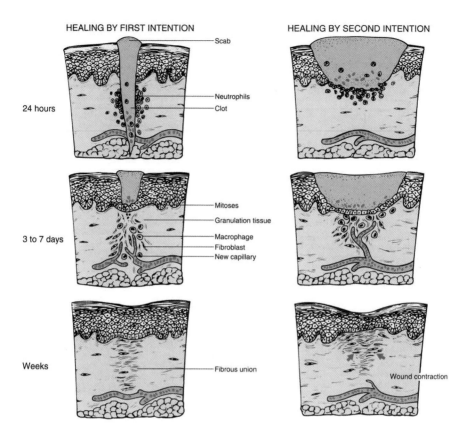

Figure 14.1 Healing by intention. (Reproduced with permission. From *Robbins Pathologic Basis of Disease*. 6th ed. Philadelphia: WB Saunders Co; 1999.)

by primary intention are associated with minimal basement membrane interruption, tissue loss, and cellular damage.

Second Intention

Second intention healing is associated with more extensive loss of tissue and unapposed wound edges. Granulation tissue is formed and subsequently connective tissue deposited. A prominent feature of healing by second intention is wound contracture, the process whereby the surrounding normal tissue is pulled toward the area of the initial wound by the scarring process.

Third Intention

Healing by third intention (also called *delayed primary intention*) entails septic wounds. Typically such a wound is debrided, treated, and left open until such time it is deemed suitable to be closed. It is important to remember that the sequence of healing events is the same regardless of the type of wound.

THE PROCESS OF HEALING

The process of wound healing has classically been divided into three phases: inflammation, proliferation, and tissue maturation. These stages are not mutually exclusive. They are a continuum of events, and all three stages may occur simultaneously. Vascular tissue injury causes bleeding that initiates a hemostatic response. In the inflammatory phase, neutrophils infiltrate and protect the site from microbes and begin the process of cleaning up necrotic tissue and cells. Macrophages continue the role of debridement, but also secrete factors that initiate the proliferative phase. In this phase, fibroblasts begin secreting connective tissue proteins. Vascular endothelial cells initiate the process of angiogenesis. Epithelial cells migrate over the wound surface and myofibroblasts, through cell-matrix interactions, contract the wound and facilitate wound closure. In the maturational stage, fibroblasts continue to secrete the structural proteins and proteases necessary for the reorganization of collagen fibrils; both aid in increasing wound strength and tissue flexibility. The process of wound healing varies in different ocular tissues.

The length of time needed for wound healing depends on many factors, including tissue vascularity, availability of chemoattractant factors, and cellular proliferation rates. In general, the more vascular the tissue the quicker it tends to heal, as increased vascularity allows for not only a more robust cellular response, but also can support greater cellular proliferation. Because regulating the vascularity of a tissue without causing injury is more complex, modulation of wound healing is often accomplished by diminishing and slowing cellular response and proliferation mechanisms. For instance, the skin of the face is usually sutured with nylon monofilaments. These minimize localized cellular response at the wound site, helping to prevent scarring. Similarly, medications such as steroids can be used to slow the cellular response or the proliferation of certain cells in deference to others. As you will see, these techniques are applied to tissues differentially depending on the demands of the wound healing process, and techniques vary from tissue to tissue.

WOUND HEALING IN DERMAL/CONJUNCTIVAL TISSUE

Conjunctiva and dermis both are highly vascular tissues with like cellular and stromal structure and similarity in wound healing issues.

Inflammatory Phase

When tissue injury occurs, the inflammatory stage of wound repair begins. The injury often involves vascular damage, leading to the extravasation of blood into soft tissues. Tissue hemostasis involves an orchestration of many cellular components including vascular endothelial cells, platelets, and the coagulation cascade. It is important to appreciate that the initial clot structure that fills the wound space has functions in addition to simple hemostasis. The newly formed structure is rich in fibrin and glycoproteins that facilitate binding of cellular adhesion molecules necessary for cellular migration. The clot also serves as a storage site for various growth factors that were either trapped from blood components or secreted from cells at the wound site. This reservoir sets up a concentration gradient that further aids in directing cellular migration and wound repair.

Many of the protein factors involved in the coagulation cascade also play a role in stimulating inflammation. The kinin enzymatic cascade directly triggers the complement system, producing anaphylatoxins that are strong mediators of inflammation. An end product of the kinin pathway, bradykinin, increases vascular permeability and vasodilatation. The endothelium secretes enzymes that degrade the fibrin clot into various fragments called *split products* or *fibrin degradation products*, which are chemotactic for neutrophils. They also act together to induce monocyte and neutrophil adhesion and migration toward the complement components at the site of healing. Early in the process, neutrophils are recruited to the site of damage and provide important functions including debridement and microbe control at the wound site by ingesting foreign bacteria, antigens, necrotic tissue, and nonviable cells.

Macrophages play a central role in wound healing, arriving hours after the inflammatory response begins. The circulating precursors to macrophages, monocytes are recruited to the wound location by various chemoattractants, where they mature into macrophages. As well as being proinflammatory, macrophages are crucial to tissue debridement by clearing any residual bacteria, necrotic tissue, and senescent neutrophils. Macrophages synthesize proteases capable of degrading a wide range of extracellular matrix constituents. Several of the zinc-dependent matrix metalloproteinases (MMPs) are synthesized as well. MMPs are important for many biologic functions, including cell migration, angiogenesis, and extracellular matrix (ECM) breakdown; they are also important to latter stages of tissue remodeling in the healing process.

Proliferative Phase

The formation of granulation tissue is a hallmark of the proliferative stage. It is marked histologically by the presence of invading fibroblasts and vascular endothelial cells. The lattice structure of the clot formed during the initial stages of hemostasis provides important binding sites for the migration of fibroblasts and new vessels. Key to wound healing, fibroblast activation elicits a multitude of responses, including secretion of growth factors, synthesis of connective tissue proteins, and expression of receptors for growth factors. The fibroblasts begin to secrete ECM proteins and ground substance components. The ECM is composed mainly of collagen, reticular and elastin fibers. Wound healing relies upon proper synthesis and deposition of collagen, and wound mechanical strength corresponds with the amount of collagen in the wound.

Fibroblasts are attracted to the initial site of injury by molecules released from platelet granules and inflammatory cells. Platelet derived growth factor (PDGF) is an important regulator of fibroblast function. Synthesis of PDGF is induced in response to factors commonly present in the wound environment such as low tissue partial pressures of oxygen, thrombin or by other cytokines and growth factors. PDGF functions as a potent chemoattractant and mitogen for fibroblasts and has been shown to stimulate protein synthesis of many matrix proteins such as collagen, fibronectin, and hyaluronic acid. It also induces synthesis of MMPs. During times of inflammation, fibroblasts and other connective tissue cells upregulate expression of the PDGF receptor.

Angiogenesis

Angiogenesis is essential in normal wound healing and occurs through a series of orderly events. The first step is activation of the endothelial cell, which entails the secretion of proteolytic enzymes. Two important proteolytic enzyme groups are the tissue plasminogen activator (t-PA)/plasmin system and the MMPs. Endothelial cells behind the leading edge of migration begin to proliferate. Normal endothelial cells do not undergo mitosis, but after injury or angiogenic stimulation they enter the cell cycle and begin division. The exact regulators of the endothelial cell cycle are not known, but it is thought that factors discussed below, which initiate neovascularization, also stimulate the endothelial cell to enter mitosis.

All of the processes necessary for formation of new vessels are mediated by a wide range of angiogenic agonists, including growth factors, chemokines, angiogenic enzymes, endothelial specific receptors, and adhesion molecules. While many factors have been documented to be angiogenic, evidence points to the potent role of vascular epithelial growth factor (VEGF) in angiogenesis. Although secreted by many cell lines, the VEGF receptor is for the most part restricted to the endothelial cells. VEGF is a chemoattractant and mitogen to vascular endothelium, guiding new vessel formation.

Epithelialization

The most basic function of the epithelial layer is to protect the organism from environmental insults. Between adjacent epithelial cell membranes are specialized adhesion proteins that form occluding or tight junctions. Additionally, epithelial cells are anchored to a basement membrane; this layer contains many of the same components as the extracellular matrix but has a predominance of type IV collagen, laminin, and heparan sulfate. In wound healing, basement membrane provides adhesion sites and migratory signals to proliferating cells.

After injury, it is imperative for the epithelium to seal off the wound from the external environment. In order to accomplish this, existing epithelial cells must disassociate from anchoring fibers and migrate over the matrix of the initial clot in the wound. Additionally, if basement membrane continuity is disrupted, it must be replaced. Growth factors have also been implicated in inducing the migratory and proliferative responses of epithelial cells after injury. Just as VEGF plays a major role in angiogenesis, the tear film component epithelial growth factor (EGF) is a key regulator of migration and proliferation of epithelial cells of all types, and evidence points to the lacrimal gland as a synthesizer of these molecules.

Wound Contraction

In conjunction with re-epithelialization, contraction of the wound helps close and decrease its size. Substantial evidence points to a differentiated form of fibroblast, the myofibroblast, as the cause of contraction. Within granulation tissue, these altered cells acquire features typical of smooth muscle, including cytoplasmic expression of microfilaments composed of myosin and α-smooth muscle actin.

Tissue Maturation Phase

The tissue maturation phase of healing is characterized by the modification of the granulation tissue into a scar combined with a decrease in cellularity of the scar. Components of the granulation tissue begin to transform from the initial fibrin- and fibronectin-rich network deposited in the wound site at the initial stages to a collagen-rich scar tissue. Remodeling of the wound tissue is a net result of a degradative versus synthetic process. As reflected earlier, the synthetic processes are carried out chiefly through the actions of the fibroblast. The degradative processes are influenced heavily by the enzymatic actions of MMPs and their endogenous inhibitors (tissue inhibitors of metalloproteinases, sometimes called TIMPs). Research is now beginning to show that overaction of MMPs leads to prolonged wound healing and importantly scarring through excessive ECM destruction. New research, in vitro, involving a synthetic MMP inhibitor has shown significant results for decreasing collagen production and fibroblast-collagen matrix contraction. In vivo studies in animal models show that MMP inhibition significantly increases bleb survival time and maintains postoperative intraocular pressure and bleb area. Remodeling can begin early at the wound edges and can continue for months. While the fibrin clot is being degraded, collagen and other proteins are being synthesized and deposited in the wound site.

Practical Considerations

Wound healing in conjunctiva and dermis can be accomplished by either primary or secondary intention. In general, primary closure allows for more controlled healing and is used on the skin of the face and exposed conjunctiva. This type of wound closure is preferable as it minimizes scarring, while healing by secondary intention takes much longer and often leaves more prominent scars. Nonetheless, healing by secondary intention may be useful in cases of anterior segment reconstruction or reconstructive oculoplastic surgery. For instance, healing by secondary intention is often applied after the removal of conjunctival and/or dermal tumors in which a large graft is needed, and the wound cannot be closed by primary intention.

The average time to re-epithelialization of conjunctiva and facial skin is quite short, on the order of several days. By postoperative day 5, the edges of most skin incisions will have re-epithelialized. However, wounds of the facial skin may require attention for longer periods in order to prevent scar formation. For instance, sutures in facial skin are usually removed in 5 to 7 days in order to avoid an inflammatory reaction to the suture material. The wound only has 10% of its tensile strength at this time and usually requires at least an additional week of suppression of the cellular response in order to avoid scar formation. Supplemental support (eg, steri-strips) may be required to maintain tissue apposition.

Wounds of the facial skin achieve greater than 50% tensile strength within about 2 weeks, 70% to 80% by 3 months. Conjunctival wounds achieve similar strengths in nearly half the time. The choice of suture material, as well as type of suture placed, alter the way in which the tissue heals. Generally, nonorganic nylon monofilaments are used on the skin of the face in order to minimize chemoattraction. Topical steroids are then often used to further slow the cellular response. Whereas these measures also slow cellular proliferation to a certain extent, causing the wound to heal slower, the decreased cellular response produces a more-favorable outcome. Conjunctival closures, in which a more robust cellular response is generally desired, usually utilize Vicryl or gut sutures. These create a greater cellular response at the wound site, allowing for faster healing and increased tensile strength in a shorter time, as well as increased scar formation.

The short period to re-epithelialization can be problematic in cases where the wound was improperly constructed or where the wound margins were unapposed. The intervening gap will now heal by secondary intention, causing a visible scar. In these cases, wounds must be revised by creating "fresh" margins and re-apposing them. Removal of any granulation tissue must also be accomplished as this will speed healing and avoid cyst formation. If this removal is not possible, there must be minimal disturbance of the granulation tissue in order to prevent scarring. This can be achieved through the use of topical steroid/antibiotic combinations, but at the cost of very prolonged healing time.

During a glaucoma filtration surgery, special care to achieve hemostasis is required. We have learned that residual bleeding and clots can spur early bleb failure by acting as a source and reservoir for many inflammatory components.

CORNEAL WOUND HEALING

The healthy cornea is devoid of vessels; therefore, corneal stromal wound healing is characterized by the absence of a vascular stage. Instead of granulation tissue, there is formation of fibroblastic tissue, a similar tissue without blood vessels. The corneal stroma has three major components: proteoglycans, keratocytes, and collagen, predominantly type I. When corneal tissue is damaged, fibrin and fibronectin aggregate at the wound. Fibrin derives from anterior chamber exudates in penetrating wounds, limbal vessels, and conjunctival vessels; keratocytes produce fibronectin. These elements are essential for cellular migration, proliferation, and collagen remodeling. Keratocytes are essential cells in the healing process and perform multiple functions depending on the chemical messengers in the stroma, including actions as fibroblasts, myofibroblasts, and phagocytic cells. Fibroblasts, keratocytes, and monocytes may show fibroblastic behaviors as well as phagocytic activity. Neutrophils are involved in phagocytosis of dead cells and damaged stromal constituents as well as defend against infection. Cells with fibroblastic activity deposit proteoglycans and collagen fibrils, forming a scar. The stromal scar is remodeled, with constituency becoming more like healthy tissue with time. However, the scar may never have the same tensile strength as surrounding healthy tissue.

Epithelial cell wound healing involves multiple phases, including sliding of superficial cells, cell mitosis, and stratification for normal epithelial anatomy. Should the wound involve Bowman's layer and superficial stroma, the epithelium will fill in the extra space, forming an epithelial facet; Bowman's layer and superficial stroma are not regenerated. Epithelial anchoring to the underlying stroma is rapid when a basement membrane is present; anchoring is significantly delayed if the basement membrane was ablated. Cell migration begins at approximately 5 hours after injury at 60 to 80 μm per hour. Intact epithelium increases the tensile strength of the underlying stroma, but an epithelial plug may prevent healing of a stromal wound.

Ablation of corneal tissue using an excimer laser induces a healing response as well. Initially epithelial cells migrate and proliferate over the wound bed using collagen, fibronectin, and various glycoproteins as described earlier in this chapter. Re-epithelialization of the wound bed usually is complete within a few days. Stromal reaction to ablation follows that of connective tissue in general. There is a migration, proliferation, and activation of stromal keratocytes that begin to secrete collagen, glycoproteins, and various components of the ECM. In time, the anterior stromal surface achieves a relatively normal lamellar appearance.

Following refractive keratotomy procedures, the corneal epithelium migrates and proliferates into the wound, forming an unpredictably persistent epithelial plug that initially retards normal wound healing. This plug has been shown to persist for up to 70 months in incision sites, but the corneal basement membrane with all of its attachments ultimately regenerates. After the initial stromal inflammatory response with edema, the keratocytes ultimately fill the plug with connective tissue forming two distinct morphologically variable scars. These two types of scars have described as either thin, with feathery edges extending from the incision site, or as rougher and broad with an increased width containing epithelial inclusions.

Following full-thickness incisions or lacerations, collagen and Descemet's membrane retract due to their inherent elasticity. Fibrin and fibronectin fill the wound space providing a scaffold for migrating cells. As migrating epithelium

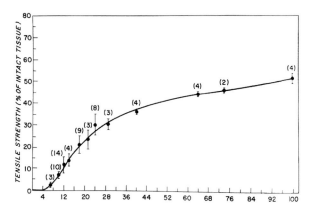

Figure 14.2 Tensile strength of healing central corneal wounds expressed in percentage of value for intact tissue. The numbers in parenthesis are error scores. (Reproduced with permission. From Gasset AR, Dohlman CH. The tensile strength of corneal wounds. *Arch Ophthalmol.* 1968;79:595–602.)

fills the wound site, proper care should be given to appose the wound edges to prevent epithelial down growth. A stromal reaction ensues with production of ECM by fibroblasts. The endothelium heals in a similar manner to that described for all epithelial tissue. Initially, there is a migration of cells over the wound site. If there is compromise of the basement membrane, in this case Descemet's membrane, there is synthesis of a new one.

Due to the avascular nature of the cornea, incisional wounds tend to heal slowly. Animal models show that central corneal wounds with respect to time have less than 5% tensile strength compared to that of intact tissue at 1 week and 45% at 2 months time (Figure 14.2). Also of importance is the fact that a denuded cornea significantly slowed underlying stromal healing, demonstrated by a delay in gain of tensile strength as compared to wounded nondenuded corneas. Highlighting the importance of vascular supply with respect to speed of healing is the fact that corneoscleral wounds showed 14% to 24% tensile strength to that of intact tissue at 1 week and by 6 weeks the wound strength was recorded at 50% that of intact tissue.

Practical Considerations

Due to the nature of the tissue and its anatomic function, healing by primary intention (suture or glue closure) is required in full- and partial-thickness corneal wounds. Epithelial injury, however, is usually left to heal by secondary intention since the epithelial cells migrate over denuded areas in a very short period. In fact, most epithelial injury is fully healed in 72 hours.

As previously mentioned, the avascular nature of the cornea is the single greatest obstacle to wound healing in this tissue. Therefore, the surgeon must account for this fact in the choice of suture and technique. For instance, central corneal wounds can take months to achieve even 50% tensile strength; there-fore, semipermanent sutures are placed in order to maintain wound integrity during this prolonged period. Once again, in order to minimize scar forma-tion (the cornea must remain clear), nylon monofilaments are used as they will minimize any cellular response. Topical steroids are again used to further retard cellular response. This process will take several months. Interestingly enough, corneal epithelial healing seems to be only minimally retarded by steroid use in an otherwise healthy cornea. The same is not true of anesthetic corneas where lack of neurotropic factors retards epithelial healing. In these instances steroid use must be modulated to avoid complications. Experimen-tally, the use of nerve growth factor has shown promise as a means of re-epithelialization without altering the cellular response.

The technique with which the sutures are applied is also important in wound contracture modulation. Given the circular nature of most central cor-neal wounds as well as the anatomic curvature of the cornea, the use of inter-rupted sutures is necessary in order to be able to modify the wound contrac-ture to avoid astigmatism.

SCLERAL WOUND HEALING

Scleral tissue heals by the formation of granulation tissue despite its relatively few native vessels. Depending on the anatomic site of injury, the sclera derives the cellular constituents needed for healing from nearby vascular components. Superficial scleral injury engages the overlying episcleral vessels, and if the inner sclera is compromised, the underlying choroidal vessels contribute. A perforating injury results in granulation tissue derived from both vascular sources.

Pertinent to the issue of scleral wound healing is the topic of strabismus surgery. Animal studies have shown that after muscle surgery there is an initial lag phase for approximately 4 to 5 days, followed by a linear increase in tensile strength of the musculoscleral junction. By day 8, a tensile strength of 300 grams (well over the tension produced by the muscle in extreme lateral gaze of 100 grams) was found in both recession and resection surgeries.

Practical Considerations

Once again due to the nature and function of the sclera, healing by primary intention is necessary. Scleral wounds, similar to corneal wounds, require longer healing time due to the relative avascularity of the tissue. In the sclera, however, prevention of scar formation is less important, as clarity of the tissue is not important. Nonetheless, wound contracture and cellular response must be mitigated as they can affect visual outcome.

The choice of suture material is mandated by the relatively avascular nature of the tissue, but only in part; the size and anatomic location of the scleral wound determines which material to use. For instance, the small scleral wounds created in the pars plana during vitrectomy are usually closed with Vicryl sutures. The absorbable material increases cellular response at the wound site and speeds the repair process. In this case, there is no underlying retina, and the danger of neovascularization is minimal. In contrast, more posterior scleral wounds, such as those seen in ruptured globe cases, must be closed with nonabsorbable nylon monofilaments. In these cases, tensile strength is paramount. It may take sclera several months to achieve 50% tensile strength, and the tissue may never achieve the same tensile strength as the surrounding uninjured tissue. Therefore, there is an increased risk of rupture at this site. In addition, the choroid underlies these wounds and the nylon monofilaments minimize the risk of neovascularization.

Strabismus surgery presents a different aspect of scleral healing. The musculoscleral wounds in these surgeries heal at a much faster rate due to the highly vascularized muscle. The vascularity of the muscle provides a desirable increased cellular response which speeds healing; the process also may be increased by the use of absorbable suture material (Vicryl). However, the fact that healing times are not significantly prolonged by use of the "hang back" technique (in which the suture is merely a place holder) as compared to the "crossed swords" technique (in which the muscle is tightly reapposed to the scleral insertion) would seem to indicate that the presence of suture material minimally influences cellular response in these cases.

UVEAL WOUND HEALING

While the ciliary body and choroid heal through deposition of granulation tissue and subsequent scar formation, the iris behaves in a different manner. The anatomy of the iris lesion dictates whether healing takes place. A lesion oriented in a perpendicular fashion to that of the radial fibers allows the radial muscles to pull the wound edges apart, gaping the wound. Wound healing does not extend across the gap. A lesion oriented parallel to the radial fibers leaves the wound edges closely approximated. Subsequently, iris epithelium begins to migrate to cover the wound and stroma begins to secrete collagen fibrils and ground substance.

MODIFYING WOUND HEALING

Scarring of any ocular tissue can result in decreased vision and a subsequent increase in patient morbidity. Current research includes methods to modify the steps of wound healing to reduce poor visual outcomes.

Suture Materials

A simple means of modifying wound healing is in the choice of suture materials. If more rapid healing is desired, then sutures capable of inducing an inflammatory reaction are used. These include Vicryl, gut, and silk. If inflammation is not desirable, monofilament sutures such as Prolene and nylon may be used. In some surgeries it may be desirable to do both. For example, in a limbal-based trabeculectomy, nylon sutures are used to close the scleral flap, as inflammation and scarring in this area are undesirable, inhibiting aqueous flow around the flap. However, when closing the conjunctiva, a Vicryl suture is used to encourage inflammation at the incision site to promote scarring and a watertight closure. Table 14.1 compares suture materials. Also see Chapter 6 for additional information.

Table 14.1. Comparison of Suture Materials and Properties

Example	Material	Filament	Cellular Response	Absorbable	Time to Resorption
Gut (plain)	Bovine intestine	monofilament	Marked	Yes	5–7 days
Gut (chromic)	Bovine intestine	monofilament	Marked	Yes	2–3 weeks
Mersilene	Polyethylene terephthalate	braided	Mild	No	N/A
Nylon	Nylon	mono- or multifilament	None–mild	No	N/A
Prolene	Polypropylene	monofilament	None–mild	No	N/A
Silk	Silk	braided	Mild–moderate	No	N/A
Vicryl	Polyglactin	braided (monofilament available)	Moderate	Yes	6–8 weeks

Currently, experimentation with light-activated, scaffold-enhanced protein solder and commercially available bioadhesives such as cyanoacrylate has shown promise for future use. Bioadhesives may even be able to replace sutures in some cases, possibly providing faster surgical times, lower risks, and improved healing times. Tissue glue may in the future be used in clear cornea cataract cases and decrease risk of endophthalmitis.

Anti-Inflammatories

The administration of corticosteroids reduces postoperative inflammation, affecting all stages of wound healing. In the acute stages, they interfere with neutrophil adherence to vessel walls and migration. Later in the process, they inhibit the formation of plasmin through action on plasminogen activators, thereby preventing degradation of fibrin, whose products aid in recruitment of neutrophils, and preventing activation of MMPs. They further impair inflammation by lymphocytolysis.

Nonsteroidal anti-inflammatory drugs (NSAIDs) have been shown to inhibit some cell adhesion interactions in the early stages of inflammation. NSAIDs nonspecifically inhibit the isoforms of cyclooxygenase, the enzyme necessary for the transformation of arachidonic acid into prostaglandins, vasoactive substances that indirectly facilitate leukocyte migration. More recent studies have shown that topical NSAIDs may have a negative effect on normal corneal wound healing, by destroying newly deposited ECM, through the induction of early synthesis of MMPs by corneal epithelium.

Antiproliferative Agents

The use of antiproliferative agents is the current gold standard in glaucoma filtration surgery to delay postsurgical scarring. The two most common agents are 5-fluorouracil (5-FU) and mitomycin C. 5-FU is a pyrimidine analog that inhibits RNA synthesis through its conversion to 5'-uridine monophosphate (5-UMP) and its subsequent incorporation into the mRNA. DNA synthesis is inhibited through its conversion to deoxyuridine 5' phosphate, which inhibits thymidylate synthesis. Mitomycin C, an antibiotic, inhibits DNA synthesis through its ability to cross link DNA molecules and induce single-strand breaks.

While these therapies have improved the success of glaucoma surgeries, limitations remain. While single exposure to antiproliferatives impairs fibroblast replication, it does not stop them from secreting growth factors, expressing growth factor receptors, and producing ECM matrix molecules.

Current research is investigating the effects of either supplementing or blocking these growth factors. Intravitreal injections of basic fibroblast growth factor in rabbits significantly increased photoreceptor survival and restoration of the blood–retinal barrier after argon laser injury over that of controls. Applications of anti-TGF-β2 antibody in glaucoma filtration surgery in rabbits significantly reduced fibroblast number, wound contraction, and increased bleb survival time. Administration of cyclosporine A, an immunosuppressive agent, led to a decrease in wound healing parameters. EGF applied topically to traumatic corneal abrasions yielded a significant improvement in epithelial healing time. VEGF inhibitors may find use in other subspecialties than retina, possibly in wound modulation of glaucoma surgeries. Possible future therapies include modification of gene expression, antisense oligonucleotides, gene transfers, neutralizing monoclonal antibodies, and ribozymes. It is likely that a "cocktail" of therapeutic agents, targeting different components of the wound healing process to optimize surgical outcomes, will be the standard of care.

THE ULTIMATE GOAL

In summary, this chapter has sought to provide a solid base of knowledge on the healing process. Young ophthalmologists who are the future of the field are challenged to spur novel ideas on how to modulate wound healing on the molecular level. The short- and long-term goals of improving surgical outcomes coincide well with the ultimate goal of optimal patient care.

KEY POINTS

→ Wound healing by first intention involves approximation of wound edges with sutures, resulting in less scarring, while healing by secondary intention involves unapposed wound edges and granulation tissue formation, with more scarring.

→ Corneal wound healing is prolonged due to avascularity and requires permanent sutures to maintain wound approximation and prevent scarring.

→ Wound healing may be modulated by choice of suture, type of closure, anti-inflammatory, and other immunosuppressive medications.

SELF-ASSESSMENT TEST

1. Conjunctival and skin wound healing are characterized by (list all that apply)
   a. Inflammation and coagulation
   b. Invading fibroblasts and endothelial cells
   c. Angiogenesis, modulated by VEGF
   d. Epithelialization, modulated by epithelial growth factor (EGF)
   e. All of the above
2. Corneal wound healing differs from conjunctival and scleral wound healing in the following ways (list all that apply)
   a. Lack of vascular stage
   b. Neutrophils are not involved
   c. Slower healing
   d. Epithelial plugs may facilitate wound healing
3. Time to regain approximately 50% tensile strength after wound creation is (cornea vs corneoscleral)
   a. 6 weeks vs > 2 months
   b. > 2 months vs 6 weeks
   c. 1 week vs 3 weeks
   d. 3 weeks vs 1 week
4. Wound healing may be delayed by (list all that apply)
   a. Corticosteroids
   b. 5-FU
   c. Cyclosporine
   d. Absorbable suture material

For preferred responses to these questions, see pages 223–224.

SUGGESTED READING

Apt L, Gaffney WL, Dora AF. Experimental suture studies in strabismus surgery. I. Reattachment rate of extraocular muscles after recession and resection operations. *Albrecht Von Graefes Arch Klin Exp Ophthalmol.* 1976;201:11–17.

Azar DT, Hahn TW, Khoury JM. Corneal wound healing following laser surgery. In: Azar DT, ed. *Refractive Surgery.* Stamford, CT: Appleton & Lange; 1997:41–62.

Bowman PH, Fosko SW, Hartstein ME. Periocular reconstruction. *Semin Cutan Med Surg.* 2003;22:263–272.

Chabner BA, Ryan DP, Paz-Ares L, et al. Antineoplastic agents. In: Hardman JG, Limbird LE, Gilman AG, eds. *Goodman and Gilman's The Pharmacological Basis of Therapeutics.* 10th ed. New York: McGraw-Hill Professional; 2001:1389–1460.

Chang L, Crowston JG, Cordeiro MF, et al. The role of the immune system in conjunctival wound healing after glaucoma surgery. *Surv Ophthalmol.* 2000;45:49–68.

Cordeiro MF, Schultz GS, Ali RR, et al. Molecular therapy in ocular wound healing. *Br J Ophthalmol.* 1999;83:1219–1224.

Cordeiro MF. Beyond Mitomycin: TGF-beta and wound healing. *Prog Ret Eye Res.* 2002;21:75–89.

Cotran RS, Kumar V, Collins T. Acute and chronic inflammation. In: *Robbins Pathologic Basis of Disease.* 6th ed. Philadelphia: WB Saunders Co; 1999:50–88.

Cotran, RS, Kumar V, Collins T. Tissue repair: cellular growth, fibrosis, and wound healing. In: *Robbins Pathologic Basis of Disease.* 6th ed. Philadelphia: WB Saunders Co; 1999:89–112.

Furie B, Furie BC. The molecular basis of blood coagulation. In Hoffman R, ed. *Hematology: Basic Principles and Practice.* 3rd ed. New York: Churchill Livingstone, Inc; 2000:1783–1804.

Gasset AR, Dohlman CH. The tensile strength of corneal wounds. *Arch Ophthalmol.* 1968;79:595–602.

Hanna C, Roy FH. Iris wound healing. *Arch Ophthalmol.* 1972;88:296–304.

Hertle RW, James M, Farber MG. Insertion site dynamics and histology in a rabbit model after conventional or suspension rectus recession combined with ipsilateral antagonist resection. *J Pediatr Ophthalmol Strabismus.* 1993;30:184–191.

Hoffman GT, Soller EC, Bloom JN, et al. A new technique of tissue repair in ophthalmic surgery. *Biomed Sci Instrum.* 2004;40:57–63.

Johnston WT, Filatov V, and Talamo JH. Corneal wound healing following refractive keratotomy. In: Azar DT, ed. *Refractive Surgery.* Stamford, CT: Appleton & Lange; 1997:29–40.

Kinoshita S, Adachi W, Sotozono C, et al. Characteristics of the human ocular surface epithelium. *Prog Retin Eye Res*. 2001;20:639–673.

Kumar V, Abbass AK, Fausto N. Tissue renewal and repair: regeneration, healing, and fibrosis. In: *Robbins and Cotran's Pathologic Basis of Disease*. 7th ed. Philadelphia: WB Saunders Co; 2005:113–114.

McDermott M. Stromal wound healing. In: Brightbill FS, ed. *Corneal Surgery: Theory, Technique & Tissue*. St Louis: Mosby, Inc; 1999:40–48.

Phillips LG. Wound healing. In: Sabiston CM, ed. *Textbook of Surgery*. 16th ed. Philadelphia: WB Saunders Co; 2001:131–144.

Ribatti D, Vacca A, Presta M. The discovery of angiogenic factors: a historical review. *Gen Pharmacol*. 2000;35:233–239.

Stenn KS, Malhotra R. Epithelialization. In: Cohen KI, Diegelmann RF, Linblad WJ, eds. *Wound Healing: Biochemical & Clinical Aspects*. Philadelphia: WB Saunders Co; 1992:115–127.

Ware AJ. Cellular mechanisms of angiogenesis. Ware AJ, Simons M, eds. *Angiogenesis and Cardiovascular Disease*. New York: Oxford University Press; 1999:30–59.

Yanoff M, Fine BS. *Ocular Pathology: A Text and Atlas*. 3rd ed. Philadelphia: JB Lippincott Co; 1989:103–162.

Chapter 15

Dressings

David K. Wallace, MD

Dressings are placed at the conclusion of many ophthalmic procedures, although some surgeries do not require them, and there is a general trend to use them less frequently than in previous years. Each surgeon has his or her own preferences for the use and selection of dressings; for the same ophthalmic procedure, some surgeons will choose to use a dressing and others will not. This chapter reviews the major advantages and disadvantages of ophthalmic postoperative dressings; the major surgical procedures for which these dressings are typically used; the materials commonly used; and techniques for placement of pressure and nonpressure dressings.

ADVANTAGES AND DISADVANTAGES OF POSTOPERATIVE DRESSINGS

The advantages of postoperative dressings include

→ Absorption of blood and ocular secretions
→ Reduction of postoperative edema, especially if applied with pressure
→ Reduction of the risk of injury to the operated site, especially in children
→ In some cases, increased patient comfort (eg, in the presence of an epithelial defect)

→ Prevention of exposure keratopathy after procedures involving an eyelid block and/or retrobulbar or peribulbar anesthesia

→ In major orbital surgeries, prevention of the accumulation of fluid and blood in empty spaces (pressure dressing)

The disadvantages of postoperative dressings include

→ Patient discomfort, due to tightness, itching and/or excessive warmth

→ Possible delay of the diagnosis of complications such as infection or excessive bleeding

→ Prevention of the administration of topical medications prior to its removal

→ In some cases, delay of the healing process

→ Production of exposure keratopathy (if improperly applied)

→ Rare complications such as central retinal artery occlusion (with pressure dressings)

→ Damage to delicate eyelid tissues (if not carefully removed)

→ Skin irritation or allergic reactions from adhesive tapes

In selected cases, it may thus be preferable to defer the use of a dressing.

INDICATIONS

A dressing is typically applied after the following ophthalmic procedures:

→ Major oculoplastics procedures, including surgery of anophthalmic sockets and orbital decompression

→ Vitreoretinal surgery, including posterior vitrectomy or scleral buckle

→ Penetrating keratoplasty

→ Trabeculectomy

→ Extracapsular cataract extraction

→ Adjustable suture strabismus surgery, in order to provide comfort and to protect the sutures from dislodgment

→ Any intraocular procedure in a child

→ Any procedure for which an eyelid block and/or retrobulbar or peribulbar anesthesia is used, to prevent exposure keratopathy from lagophthalmos

→ Any procedure in which a corneal epithelial defect is created, intentionally (eg, goniotomy) or unintentionally

→ Any procedure in which a large amount of postoperative conjunctival edema is anticipated (eg, some strabismus re-operations)

A dressing is typically not applied after the following ophthalmic procedures:

→ Most minor ophthalmic plastic procedures, including ptosis surgery or minor eyelid procedures
→ Uncomplicated phacoemulsification with topical anesthesia (shield only)
→ Strabismus surgery

SUPPLIES

Table 15.1 lists the soft dressing materials, eye shields, tape, and other supplies used in applying dressings. Here are key points about these items:

→ *Telfa* is indicated as the first layer if removal of the patch could damage delicate tissues beneath it, such as skin grafts. One piece of telfa is cut to a size slightly larger than the wound or graft, and it is placed gently on the incision site (Figure 15.1).
→ *Oval eye pads* are used for most dressings. The standard technique for nonpressure or pressure dressings is outlined in the next section.

Table 15.1. Supplies for Dressings

Category	Type
Soft dressing materials	Telfa Oval eye pads Gauze
Eye shields	Adult vs child size Right vs left Plastic vs metal
Tape	Paper Silk Plastic
Other	Steri-strips Skin adhesive (eg, Mastisol)

Figure 15.1. Telfa is cut to proper size to cover a surgical incision. (Illustration by Mark M. Miller)

Telfa

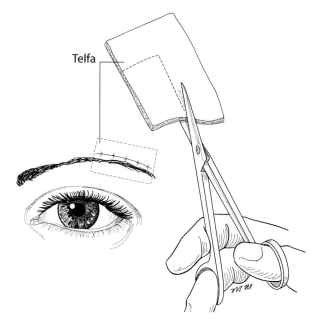

→ *Gauze* can be used as part of a large pressure dressing or in place of a dressing altogether. After some minor oculoplastics procedures, ice-soaked gauze is applied directly on the incision site immediately at the conclusion of surgery.

→ *Eye shields* can be used with or without soft dressings beneath them. They are often used without a soft dressing after uncomplicated phacoemulsification with topical anesthetic. They are sometimes used at night only to prevent unintentional injury to the operative site from unconscious rubbing of it.

→ *Tape* is available in many materials, including paper, silk, plastic, and Elastoplast. Paper tape is extremely lightweight and generally causes less skin irritation than other types. Silk and plastic tapes are stronger than paper tape and are more easily torn into pieces with square edges. Elastoplast can be used when a large amount of pressure is required to the surgical site.

→ *Steri-strips* are sometimes used with a skin adhesive and without a dressing for minor oculoplastics procedures to reduce wound tension.

TECHNIQUE FOR DRESSING PLACEMENT

If the decision is made to use a dressing, it should be placed neatly; it is the first impression of the results of surgery for both patient and family. The tape should be clean, its pieces should be approximately the same length, and its ends should be square. Dressings are almost never placed on both eyes because of the psychological impact of bilateral occlusion. Exceptions include bilateral enucleations and bilateral intraocular surgery, sometimes performed in infants with cataracts or glaucoma.

Nonpressure Dressing With a Shield

An eye drop or ointment is usually administered just before a dressing is placed. Several (usually four or five) pieces of tape of approximately the same length are prepared ahead of time and placed in a convenient location (eg, the edge of a table) near the patient's head. An oval eye pad is oriented horizontally and placed directly above the *closed* upper eyelid. The superior end of the first piece of tape is placed on the patient's forehead, and the tape is directed inferiorly and slightly temporally through the center of the eye pad to the patient's cheek (Figure 15.2). Great care is taken not to apply downward pressure on the eye during this maneuver. The inferior edge of the tape should be placed in the middle of the cheek and not too close to the corner of the patient's mouth. The tape should not be placed over the patient's hairline, or removal postoperatively

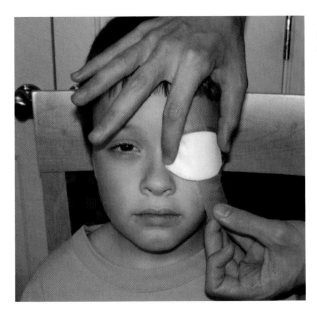

Figure 15.2. First piece of tape applied over center of eye pad.

will be difficult and painful, especially in children. Other pieces of tape are applied in a similar manner, progressively nasal and temporal to the center piece until the entire eye pad is covered (Figure 15.3). A shield that is appropriate for the patient's eye (left or right) and age (child vs adult) is then applied over the patch. A single piece of tape placed in the same orientation as the first piece placed over the eye pad is usually sufficient to secure the shield (Figure 15.4).

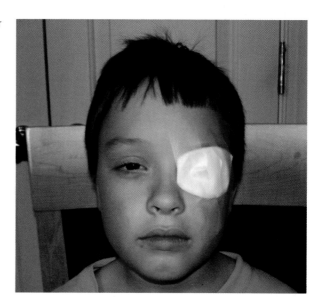

Figure 15.3. Appearance after all pieces of tape applied to soft dressing.

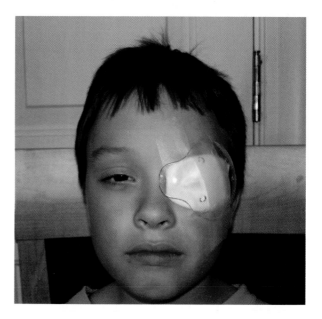

Figure 15.4. Final appearance of dressing after shield placement.

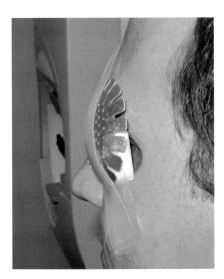

Figure 15.5. Proper placement of a shield in contact with facial bones (side view).

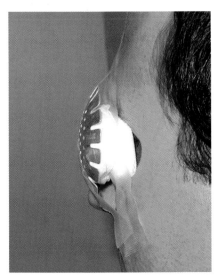

Figure 15.6. Improper placement of a shield with edges not in contact with facial bones (side view).

The edges of the shield should be in contact with the bones surrounding the orbital rim (Figure 15.5). If the edges are not in contact with these bones, then any force exerted on the exterior of the shield is transmitted directly posteriorly to the eye instead of to the facial bones (Figure 15.6).

Pressure Dressing

The technique is similar to that for a nonpressure dressing, except that with a pressure dressing, the goal is to exert significant downward pressure on the wound to prevent postoperative edema and/or hemorrhage. Two oval eye pads

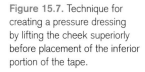

Figure 15.7. Technique for creating a pressure dressing by lifting the cheek superiorly before placement of the inferior portion of the tape.

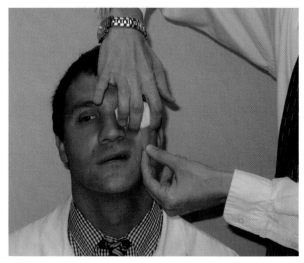

or an eye pad with gauze is used. It may be useful to have an assistant place gentle downward pressure on the dressing while the tape is placed. The maximum amount of pressure from the dressing is obtained by lifting the cheek superiorly before attaching the inferior end of each piece of tape (Figure 15.7). A skin adhesive such as Mastisol can help to seal the tape in the proper position. An eye shield is generally not needed.

POSTOPERATIVE INSTRUCTIONS

Patients should be instructed regarding the normal postoperative course, and any signs or symptoms that should prompt a call to the surgeon. When a dressing has been applied, some tightness and/or itching may be anticipated. The dressing may normally become wet with tears or blood-tinged. Patients should call if they experience excessive bleeding, pain, an unusual amount of swelling or bruising, or a fever above 101° F. In some cases, the patient may be instructed to remove the dressing on the same day as surgery. In other cases, it is left in place as long as 2 days postoperatively. If the patient is examined on the first postoperative day, the dressing will usually be removed by the surgeon or by one of the office staff.

KEY POINTS

→ Postoperative dressings protect the operative site from injury, reduce tissue fluid accumulation and absorb secretions, and may increase patient comfort.

→ Disadvantages of dressings include patient discomfort, possible delay of the diagnosis of complications such as infection or excessive bleeding, prevention of the administration of topical medications prior to its removal, and potential complications such as keratopathy, tissue damage, and allergic reactions.

→ Dressings are typically applied after procedures on children, major intraocular procedures, procedures involving eyelid or retrobulbar block, vitreoretinal surgery, and major oculoplastic procedures.

→ Major precautions for placing postoperative dressings include ensuring that the lids are closed before placing the dressing, placement of the shield so that its edges rest on the facial bones, and avoidance of excess pressure on the globe.

SELF-ASSESSMENT TEST

1. The benefits of postoperative dressings include (list all that apply)
   a. Reduction of tissue fluid accumulation
   b. Prevention of infection
   c. Protection of the operative site from injury
   d. Prevention of central retinal artery occlusion

2. The disadvantages of postoperative dressings include (list all that apply)
   a. Delayed diagnosis of complications
   b. Prevention of application of topical medications
   c. Identification of the surgical site
   d. Possible tissue damage

3. The major precautions when placing an ophthalmic postoperative dressing include (list all that apply)
   a. Be sure that no antibiotic ointment touches the cheek
   b. Ensure that the lids are closed before placing the dressing
   c. Place the shield so that its edges rest on the facial bones
   d. Avoid excess pressure on the globe while applying the dressing

4. Postoperative dressings are commonly applied after the following surgical procedures (list all that apply)

a. Trabeculectomy

b. Procedures involving eyelid or retrobulbar block

c. Bilateral strabismus surgery

d. Vitreoretinal surgery

For preferred responses to these questions, see pages 223–224.

Chapter 16

Postoperative Management

Nicholas J. Volpe, MD

The care of patients undergoing ophthalmic surgery does not end in the operating room. Provision of appropriate postoperative care and prompt, effective management of complications are critical to successful surgery. Postoperative care is the surgeon's responsibility to the patient and should not be relegated to another physician or assistant.

This chapter describes components of successful postoperative management, including

→ Communicating postoperative instructions to nursing staff and your patient
→ Scheduling timely postoperative examinations
→ Ensuring properly focused postoperative examinations
→ Recognizing and treating common complications
→ Knowing when to get assistance from others

Most patients with complications can be managed successfully with an excellent outcome if complications are recognized early and treated appropriately. These patients will require you to focus the most, because they need your expertise much more than the patient with uncomplicated surgery. Certainly these patients and the conversations you have with them must not be avoided or dispatched. You must acknowledge the "bump in the road" to your patient, be calm, and outline a careful treatment plan.

POSTOPERATIVE INSTRUCTIONS

At the conclusion of any procedure the surgeon must write appropriate orders in the patient medical record and communicate postoperative care issues and instructions to the patient and the patient's family, both verbally and in writing (Figure 16.1). Postoperative orders vary from procedure to procedure and from surgeon to surgeon. However, certain issues should be addressed in most patients:

→ Name of the procedure
→ Orders to follow the usual discharge or admission procedure of the short procedure unit
→ Instructions for body positioning and wound care
→ Antiemetic medications
→ Pain medications
→ Instructions to advance diet and discontinue intravenous fluids
→ Specific nursing instructions (eg, vision checks, use of ice, use of intravenous antibiotics)
→ Postoperative ocular medications (eg, antibiotic drops)

Patients (and family when appropriate) should hear the surgeon's initial impression as to the success of the surgery and the plan for postoperative care. This is of paramount importance to assure a good outcome. Patients must be instructed as to

→ The appropriate care of surgical wounds or dressings
→ The timing of postoperative evaluations and the application of medication
→ The type and amount of pain to be expected and how to manage it
→ Activity restrictions
→ Warning signs or symptoms requiring contact with physician and immediate attention
→ Methods and phone numbers to contact the operating surgeon

Additional issues related to postoperative care and complications vary depending on the type of procedure that was performed. Detailed discussion of specific procedures and their complications is beyond the scope of this book. However, a general discussion here focuses on the timing of postopera-

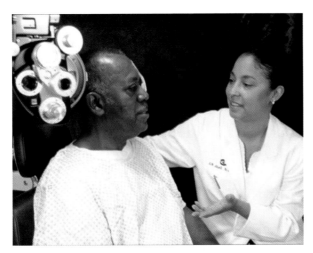

Figure 16.1. Communicating postoperative instructions to your patient—and the patient's family, if appropriate—is important to successful postoperative management. Other components are timely, focused postoperative examinations and effective management of complications. (Image courtesy National Eye Institute, National Institutes of Health)

tive care and possible complications of five broad categories of ophthalmic procedures:

→ Anterior segment surgery
→ Strabismus surgery
→ Eyelid and orbital surgery
→ Retinovitreous surgery
→ Laser surgery

TIMING OF POSTOPERATIVE CARE

The timing of appropriate postoperative care varies from procedure to procedure. Most patients are not examined on the same day of the surgery after they leave the operating room. A dressing such as an eye patch and shield are applied and then removed by the surgeon at the first follow-up visit. However there are certain circumstances in which a brief examination may be performed the same day shortly after performing the procedure. These include

→ After any type of surgery if the surgeon needs to check for recovery of motility and eyelid function after local anesthetic injection
→ After orbital or optic nerve surgery to perform vision check and rule out bleeding
→ After strabismus surgery to perform adjustment of adjustable suture
→ After laser surgeries or retinovitreous surgery with gas injection to check intraocular pressure

Specific schedules for postoperative care are determined on an individual basis determined by the surgeon and each patient's needs. The following are approximate guidelines for the five broad categories of patients.

Anterior Segment Surgery

Patients who undergo cataract surgery, glaucoma surgery, or corneal transplantation are examined for the first time on the first postoperative day. This initial examination is the most critical for ruling out unexpected intraoperative complications, measuring the initial level of visual acuity, determining the anatomic success of the procedure (eg, position of the iris or intraocular lens, depth of anterior chamber, appearance of filtration bleb, position of corneal transplant button), testing the security and water-tight nature of all surgical wounds, measuring intraocular pressure, and looking for early signs of infection. For uncomplicated cataract surgery, the subsequent examinations are generally done 1 week later and 1 month after that. Endophthalmitis generally presents between the first and seventh day postoperatively; therefore, if infection is suspected based on initial examination findings or symptoms of decreased vision, pain, or redness, sooner follow-up than 1 week would be needed. Examinations of patients undergoing filtration surgery for glaucoma are often more frequent in the first week. These patients may initially have over-filtration or leaking wounds that need to be monitored or treated (patching, bandage contact lens) or under-filtration that either needs to be watched or treated with laser suture lysis. Antimetabolites may also be used during this time. If intraocular pressure is low, careful examination for choroidal detachments is necessary. Corneal transplant patients need to be followed closely for evidence of graft failure and/or rejection that requires specific treatment.

Strabismus Surgery

Since strabismus surgery is extraocular, the risk of vision-threatening complications is lower than for intraocular procedures. Most strabismus surgeons schedule the first postoperative visit between the first day and 2 weeks after surgery. If the patient is not being seen on the first postoperative day, however, careful instructions are given to the patient or parents to call if redness or swelling develop that would suggest infection or if initial alignment of the eyes does not appear satisfactory. If adjustable sutures are used, then initial exam may be on the same day or first postoperative day for suture adjustment. For adults with multiple eye muscles operated, there is a small risk of anterior segment ischemia, and these patients are examined on the first day and in the following weeks to look for signs of this condition.

Eyelid and Orbital Surgery

Eyelid surgery patients are seen within a few days of the procedure provided there are no complaints of swelling or unexpected tenderness that would suggest infection. If adjustable suture technique is used or office modification of ptosis surgery is planned, the timing of follow-up is adjusted accordingly. Patients undergoing orbital surgery are often admitted to the hospital. Because of risk of injury to the optic nerve, ocular blood supply and adnexal structures are examined on the first postoperative day and two to three times over the following month.

Retinovitreous Surgery

The widely varying types and complexities of retinovitreous surgeries require a flexible approach to timing of postoperative evaluations. These patients are always seen on the first postoperative day and followed closely in the weeks that follow. The level of vision as well as the status of detached retina and sub-retinal fluid, intraocular gas, intraocular pressure, and presence of intraocular bleeding all determine the frequency of postoperative visits.

Laser Surgery

Laser surgery procedures are generally performed on the anterior segment for glaucoma, the cornea for refractive surgery, the posterior lens capsule for capsulotomy, and the retina for various conditions including diabetic retinopathy and choroidal neovascularization. Patients undergoing anterior segment laser procedures are often checked 1 or 2 hours after the procedure to measure intraocular pressure and one week later to determine success of the procedure. Refractive surgery patients are seen in the days after the surgery unless there are flap complications requiring more immediate attention. Patients undergoing laser surgery on the retina require follow-up at varying times in the days and weeks following the procedure, as some may require re-treatments (eg, choroidal neovascularization) and others need only be seen weeks later to determine whether treatments was successful (eg, macular treatment in diabetic retinopathy).

FOCUS OF EXAMINATION

Generally speaking, postoperative examinations are focused on determining whether the intended goal was accomplished, assessing the postoperative anatomy, looking for complications, and determining the timing of anticipated postoperative interventions such as medication changes and suture cutting. Once again the focus of the examination depends on the type of procedure performed.

Anterior Segment Surgery

The focus of this examination includes measurement of visual of acuity, determining anterior segment anatomy (intraocular lens, corneal graft or filtration bleb position), measurement of intraocular pressure, looking for intraocular inflammation (cells and flare in anterior chamber), looking for signs of infection (excessive injection, hypopyon), determination of the security of the surgical wound to be sure it is not leaking, and examination of the retina to look for perforations from anesthetic injection or retinal detachment. If visual acuity is decreased, an explanation must be found.

Strabismus Surgery

The focus of the postoperative strabismus examination is to ensure successful reattachment of muscles with normal function; to rule out scleral perforations, anterior segment ischemia, or infection; and to determine the success of the procedure. Successful strabismus surgery is characterized by maintenance of good visual acuity, successful motor alignment, and restoration of or facilitation of binocular single vision and fusion.

Eyelid and Orbital Surgery

Postoperative examination of eyelid surgery focuses on the security of skin wounds, resolution of swelling, absence of infection, and achievement of the surgical goal (eg, eyelid position in ptosis and ectropion surgery, and anatomic restoration and absence of tumor in cases of tumor excision). Postoperative evaluation after surgery for eyelid and orbital tumors must also include review of histopathology and specific diagnosis. This will help define further treatments as well as determine the adequacy of surgical margins. In patients undergoing orbital surgery, extraocular muscle function and optic nerve function should be measured.

Retinovitreous Surgery

After retinovitreous surgery, the focused examination includes a determination whether the retina is attached, holes or breaks are adequately treated, and subretinal fluid is diminished. Many procedures involve the injection of intraocular gases and the level of fill and position of the gas bubble are important considerations. Examination of the anterior segment, while lower priority, is required to assess corneal and lens clarity as well as intraocular pressure.

Laser Surgery

Laser surgery usually alters anatomy only minimally, so the postoperative examination centers on identifying secondary effects such as intraocular pressure spikes, corneal edema, and macula edema, as well as determining whether the goal of the procedure was accomplished. This involves assessment of uncorrected visual acuity in the refractive surgery patient, measurement of pressure in a patient undergoing trabeculoplasty, determination of anterior chamber depth and angle status in peripheral iridotomy patients, or adequacy of capsule opening in capsulotomy patients. The exam also assesses adequacy and extent of treatment in patients undergoing retinal laser treatment for diabetic macular edema, diabetic neovascularization (panretinal photocoagulation), and laser treatment for choroidal neovascularization. Some retinal procedures (eg, photodynamic therapy) require repeated laser applications, and in this setting the examiner must determine if re-treatment is required for continued leakage from persistent neovascularization.

PAIN MANAGEMENT

Fortunately, most patients who undergo eye surgery experience only mild to moderate pain. In fact, severe pain is often an important clue to a postoperative complication such as intraocular pressure spike, hemorrhage, or infection. Pain is generally managed with systemic medications and local maneuvers. Acetaminophen is often used as a first-line analgesic, as it is effective for mild to moderate pain and does not increase risk of hemorrhage. For more severe pain, after complications have been assessed and managed, narcotics such as codeine or oxycodone may be added. Local maneuvers include the use of ice and elevation to modify pain and swelling in patients undergoing strabismus, eyelid, or orbital surgery.

MANAGEMENT OF COMPLICATIONS

The term *complication* refers to an undesired outcome of surgery, related to an intraoperative event or a postoperative process that results in a suboptimal result. Postoperative management includes assessment for such processes and institution of measures to control the problems. It is beyond the scope of this text to detail management of specific complications; however, certain complications are more common, and assessment should include evaluation for them in each case.

Complications of Retrobulbar or Peribulbar Anesthetic Injections

Complications related to these injections include

→ Retrobulbar hemorrhage
→ Puncture of the globe
→ Injection of anesthetic into the eye
→ Injection of anesthetic into the optic nerve or subarachnoid space
→ Injection into or trauma to an extraocular muscle

Retrobulbar hemorrhage is an ophthalmic emergency. An orbital compartment syndrome can develop, and elevation of the pressure in the orbit can be severe enough to compromise ocular blood flow or raise intraocular pressure to unsafe levels. If a retrobulbar hemorrhage is encountered, the ophthalmologist must decompress the orbit by performing a lateral canthotomy and cantholysis. Puncture of the globe and/or injection of anesthetic into the eye may result in a hypotonus eye; the red reflex may appear abnormal and the anterior chamber may be deeper than normal. The puncture can lead to retinal or vitreous hemorrhage, or retinal tear or detachment. Unusual intraocular inflammation may result from the injection of anesthetic. Prompt treatment and retinovitreous surgery may be required. If the needle inadvertently is placed within the optic nerve sheath, it can cause a vision-threatening hemorrhage (sheath hematoma) requiring optic nerve sheath decompression surgery. The anesthetic can travel back to the brain and lead to seizures, respiratory depression, or cranial nerve palsies; neurologic consultation may be required for seizure control, and respiratory support may be necessary. Trauma and hemorrhage to an extraocular muscle during injection can lead to eye movement impairment and double vision; typically, no acute intervention is required, but later correction may be necessary if irreversible muscle damage occurs.

A complete list of surgical complications requiring postoperative therapy is beyond the scope of this text but some of the more common entities, along with general principles for management, are briefly described next by category.

Anterior Segment Surgery

Complications of cataract surgery include

→ Endophthalmitis, characterized by profound visual loss, severe pain, conjunctival injection, hypopyon, and vitreous opacity (vitrectomy and culture, intraocular antibiotic injection)
→ Uveitis (corticosteroid, topical and/or systemic)
→ Wound leaks (pressure patch, surgical closure)
→ Intraocular tissue prolapse through wounds (surgical replacement and closure)
→ Lost lens or lens fragments (corticosteroids, retinovitreous surgical removal)
→ Intraocular lens dislocation (surgical repositioning)
→ Elevation of intraocular pressure (pressure-lowering agents)
→ Corneal edema (manage intraocular pressure and inflammation)
→ Cystoid macular edema (topical anti-inflammatory agents)

Complications of corneal transplant surgery include

→ Graft rejection or primary graft failure (corticosteroid therapy)
→ Wound leak (surgical closure)
→ Suture abscess (suture removal if safe)
→ Persistent epithelial defects (patch, therapeutic contact lens)
→ Elevated intraocular pressure (pressure-lowering agents)

Complications of glaucoma surgery include

→ Persistence of high pressure (reinstitute medications, suture lysis, reoperation)
→ Flat or severely shallow anterior chamber secondary to overfiltration or bleb leaks (pressure patch, partial surgical closure)
→ Hyphema (pressure management; rarely, surgical evacuation)

Strabismus Surgery

Complications of strabismus surgery include

- → Over- and under-corrections (documentation, observation for stability, prisms, possible reoperation)
- → Scleral perforations (evaluation for retinal tear or detachment, retinovitreous surgery if necessary)
- → Lost or torn muscles (surgical exploration and repair)
- → Anterior segment ischemia (anti-inflammatory therapy)

Eyelid and Orbital Surgery

Complications of eyelid and orbital surgery include

- → Orbital hemorrhage (emergent cantholysis, possible orbital exploration)
- → Optic nerve damage after orbital surgery (neuroimaging to assess for bone fragments, intrasheath hemorrhage, possible reoperation for optic nerve sheath decompression)
- → Orbital cellulitis (neuroimaging to assess for abscess, systemic antibiotics, possible surgical drainage)
- → Eyelid hematoma (ice) or infection (systemic antibiotics)
- → Lagophthalmos and exposure keratitis (intensive lubricants, possible surgical repositioning)

Retinovitreous Surgery

Complications of retinovitreous surgery include

- → Failure to achieve retinal reattachment or closure of holes or tears (observe, possible reoperation)
- → Intraocular hemorrhage (observe, possible reoperation)
- → New retinal tears (re-treatment)
- → Intraocular pressure elevation, particularly when long-acting gases are used (pressure-lowering agents)

Laser Surgery

Complications of laser surgery include

→ Glaucoma laser surgery: intraocular hemorrhage, elevated intraocular pressure (pressure-lowering agents)
→ YAG capsulotomy: intraocular lens damage, intraocular pressure elevation and uveitis (pressure-lowering agents, topical corticosteroids)
→ Keratorefractive surgery: corneal flap complications (possible surgical correction), corneal infections (antibiotics)
→ Retinal laser surgery: choroidal effusions (management of intraocular pressure)

KEY POINTS

→ Postoperative counseling of the patient includes care of surgical wounds, dressings, and the application of medication, type and amount of pain to be expected, activity restrictions, and warning signs or symptoms requiring contact with physician and immediate attention.
→ At the first postoperative visit after anterior segment surgery, the examination should include determining the anatomic success of the procedure, testing the security and water tight nature of the surgical wound, measuring intraocular pressure, and looking for early signs of infection.
→ Complications of cataract surgery include endophthalmitis, uveitis, wound leaks, intraocular tissue prolapse, lost lens or lens fragments, intraocular lens dislocation, elevation of intraocular pressure, corneal edema, and cystoid macular edema.
→ Complications of strabismus surgery include over- and under-corrections, scleral perforations, lost or torn muscles, and anterior segment ischemia.

SELF-ASSESSMENT TEST

1. Postoperative counseling of the patient should include (list all that apply)
   a. Expected level of pain
   b. Activity restrictions
   c. Warning signs or symptoms requiring contact with physician and immediate attention
   d. The appropriate care of surgical wounds or dressings
   e. The timing of postoperative evaluations and the application of medication

2. For the first postoperative visit after anterior segment surgery, key features of the examination include (list all that apply)
   a. Correcting residual astigmatic error
   b. Determining the anatomic success of the procedure
   c. Testing the security and water tight nature of the surgical wound
   d. Measuring intraocular pressure
   e. Looking for early signs of infection
   f. Cleaning the posterior capsule of opacities

3. The focus of the postoperative strabismus examination is to (list all that apply)
   a. Prescribe the appropriate prism spectacle correction
   b. Remove muscle sutures
   c. Ensure successful reattachment of muscles with normal function
   d. Rule out scleral perforations, anterior segment ischemia or infection

4. Complications of retrobulbar or peribulbar anesthetic injections include (list all that apply)
   a. Retrobulbar hemorrhage
   b. Puncture of the globe
   c. Injection of anesthetic into the eye
   d. Injection of anesthetic into the optic nerve or subarachnoid space
   e. Injection into or trauma to an extraocular muscle

5. Early complications of cataract surgery include (list all that apply)
   a. Endophthalmitis
   b. Strabismus
   c. Wound leak
   d. Intraocular tissue prolapse
   e. Peripheral iridectomy
   f. Intraocular lens dislocation
   g. Elevation of intraocular pressure

For preferred responses to these questions, see pages 223–224.

Appendix A

Preferred Responses, Chapter Self-Assessment Tests

Chapter 1
1. d
2. Cardiac disease, systemic hypertension, pulmonary disease, diabetes mellitus, altered mental status
3. a, b, c

Chapter 2
1. b
2. d
3. f

Chapter 3
1. b, c, d
2. Exercise, sleep deprivation
3. True
4. a, b

Chapter 4
1. d
2. a, d
3. a, c, e, f
4. a, d

Chapter 5
1. b, c
2. a, b, d
3. b, d
4. b, c, d

Chapter 6
1. a, b
2. a, b, d
3. a, c
4. a, c, d

Chapter 7
1. a, b, c, d
2. b, c
3. a, b, d, e
4. a, b, c, d

Chapter 8
1. a, b
2. b, d
3. b
4. a, c
5. d

Chapter 9
1. True
2. a
3. False
4. d
5. d
6. True
7. True

Chapter 10
1. Hyaluronic acid
2. a, c
3. a
4. a, b, c, d
5. Identify vitreous strands, protect lens in penetrating keratoplasty, facilitate iridectomy, prevent iris capture of intraocular lens

Chapter 11
1. d
2. Excessive egress of viscoelastic and irrigating fluid, iris prolapse
3. (1) Perpendicular to the scleral surface, of approximately 50% to 60% depth, (2) parallel to scleral surface, carried anterior into clear cornea, (3) perpendicular to scleral surface at intraocular entry point
4. Corneal thermal injury, iris prolapse, postoperative iris atrophy

Chapter 12
1. b, d
2. b, c
3. a
4. a, b, d

Chapter 13
1. a, c, d
2. a
3. a, d
4. Excessive postoperative inflammation, sterile hypopyon in diabetics, intravenous infusion may be lethal
5. Increased infusion pressure, gas bubble infusion

Chapter 14
1. e
2. a, c
3. b
4. a, b, c

Chapter 15
1. a, c
2. a, b, d
3. b, c, d
4. a, b, d

Chapter 16
1. a, b, c, d, e
2. b, c, d, e
3. c, d
4. a, b, c, d, e
5. a, b, c, d, f, g

Index

Page numbers followed by *f* denote figures; those followed by *t* denote tables.

Notes